— THE GREAT —
GUT
EXTINCTION

BRENDA WATSON, CNC
WITH DR. JEMMA SINCLAIRE
AND BRENDA VALEN, BS, CNC, CNHP

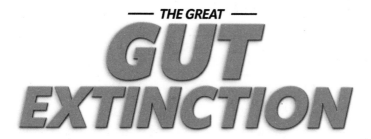

THE GREAT
GUT EXTINCTION

BRENDA WATSON, CNC
WITH DR. JEMMA SINCLAIRE
AND BRENDA VALEN, BS, CNC, CNHP

Book Design: Paul Pavlovich
Book Cover Design: Saša Bralic

Printed in the United States of America

ISBN 978-0-578-97948-9

First Printing

Brenda Watson Media
133 Candy Lane
Palm Harbor, FL 34683

ACKNOWLEDGMENTS

The gratitude I have for all the wonderful team here at Vital Planet for their help in the creation of this book is overwhelming. I have spent three decades in the natural health segment and I feel very blessed to continue to work daily with a close team of the most dedicated and creative people. We continue to produce and disseminate valuable digestive health solutions not only for humans but also for our furry family members that bring so much joy and love to our lives. I'm constantly inspired by the ongoing research that confirms that the digestive system is the true core of our overall health.

I started teaching about digestive health when science was on the brink of inquiring into gut function and how it impacted health overall. Thirty years ago in general medical circles, this was a foreign concept. My dedication and interest stemmed from my personal history of gut-related health problems. As I experienced healing success in my own body, it sparked my desire to help others realize that their gut was a huge factor in many issues of unwellness. I observed in my practice at the time, and consistently through the years since that when a person's digestive system is returned to a healthy state their overall health improved dramatically.

Always a dog lover, as I interacted with the brilliant veterinarian, Dr. Joel Murphy, I learned that our pets experience the same health problems we do. We have since been able to assist the beloved four-leggeds, which has just added to my happiness. Eternal gratitude to Dr. Murphy!

It is an ongoing crusade to contribute this restorative information to the world with books like "The Great Gut Extinction" which I believe will guide millions of people on their road to better health as they begin to understand and support their digestive systems.

For the creation of this very important book, I must thank the following people. I cherish how we work together as a diverse team and am always amazed by the creativity that naturally flows from this diversity.

First I must thank my husband Stan Watson for leading me back to the path of helping others to experience a better and more vibrant life. I never thought I would be writing another book, however his support "turned the lights on"and showed me that my career spent educating people was not over. For this, I am forever grateful.

A very special thanks to Dr. Jemma Sinclaire and her contribution to not only helping write the book and keeping us all on track but her dedication to creating a work that I as well as Vital Planet can be proud of. Without Jemma, this book would never have been brought to fruition.

Many thanks to Brenda Valen who has been beside me for 20 years in all my endeavors. She is brilliant and talented in so many ways. One of those is her ability to edit for clarity and accuracy, and for that, we are truly grateful.

Without beautiful graphics, this book could not bring the message to people in a way they could easily understand. My special thanks to the fantastic graphic artist, Paul Pavlovich, who has worked with us with passion and enthusiasm for many years on all of my book projects.

Also, we need to thank Saša Bralic for his contribution to both graphics and design of the book cover.

To my special family Chris, Joy, Ella, and Ava, I thank you for your support as we build a company dedicated to helping our world and this planet be a better place.

A very big "Thank You" to everyone at Vital Planet for your passion and persistence in getting our message out to the world. Together we will continue to strive to offer a message of digestive health to every household on this planet. I am forever amazed at the level of dedication each of you brings to Vital Planet every day!

Please enjoy this wonderful book, written by an inspired and committed team of people. With information like this, we can change the world.

Sincerely,

Brenda Watson

Brenda Watson

BIO

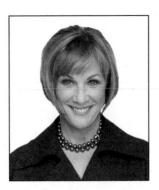

Brenda Watson, CNC

Otherwise known as the "Diva of Digestion," Brenda Watson is an amazingly successful digestive health and probiotic expert, female entrepreneur, product formulator, New York Times best-selling author, PBS celebrity, lecturer, and educator. For the last 25+ years, Brenda has dedicated her career to helping people achieve vibrant, lasting health and vitality through improved gut health and is among the foremost authorities in America today on optimum nutrition, digestive function, and natural detoxification.

As a pioneer in modern gut health, Brenda started out studying many philosophies of health and natural healing with the premier teachers of our time which inspired her to establish several natural cleansing and detoxification healthcare clinics in Florida. As Brenda continued to immerse herself in the field of digestive health, she became a master product formulator, lecturer, and educator. Knowing she had to reach more people with her message, she became an author and PBS celebrity.

To this day, Brenda has written a dozen eye-opening books and produced several successful public television specials on achieving optimal health through better digestive function. Brenda brings relevant information to the forefront in a concise and easy to understand manner, offering guideposts to vibrant health along the way.

In this latest book, Brenda delves into the newest science on the gut microbiome and the loss of microbial diversity, how it's adversely affecting our health, and what we can do about it.

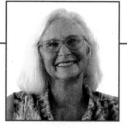

Jemma Sinclaire, D.C.

A chiropractic physician and nutritionist by trade, Jemma Sinclaire has dedicated her adult life to being helpful and supportive of healing on all levels. After, and ironically, a spinal injury limited her ability to practice chiropractic she turned her attention to her second loves, research and writing.

Meeting Brenda Watson in 2010 was a turning point in her life. Jemma's in-depth understanding of human neurology, anatomy, and physiology has proved invaluable in assisting Brenda with her last five books as well as her very popular public television shows revolving around human gut health and overall wellbeing.

Jemma's sincere hope is that whoever reads this book learns something that will light up their awareness regarding the intimate relationship of gut health to a happy life!

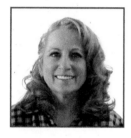

Brenda Valen, B.S., CNC, CNHP

Brenda Valen has spent a long, rewarding career in the natural products industry helping others achieve vibrant health from the inside out.

For the past two decades she has been known as "The Other Brenda," working closely with Brenda Watson on all of her books and PBS specials, and supporting her on every project. Her roles have transformed with each new situation.

As though she wasn't busy enough, Brenda has operated a health food store in Florida alongside her husband Jeff since 2013, offering diverse natural products along with cutting edge laboratory testing.

Brenda's functions continue to expand and she looks forward to many future opportunities to share the possibilities of gut health with the world!

TABLE OF **CONTENTS**

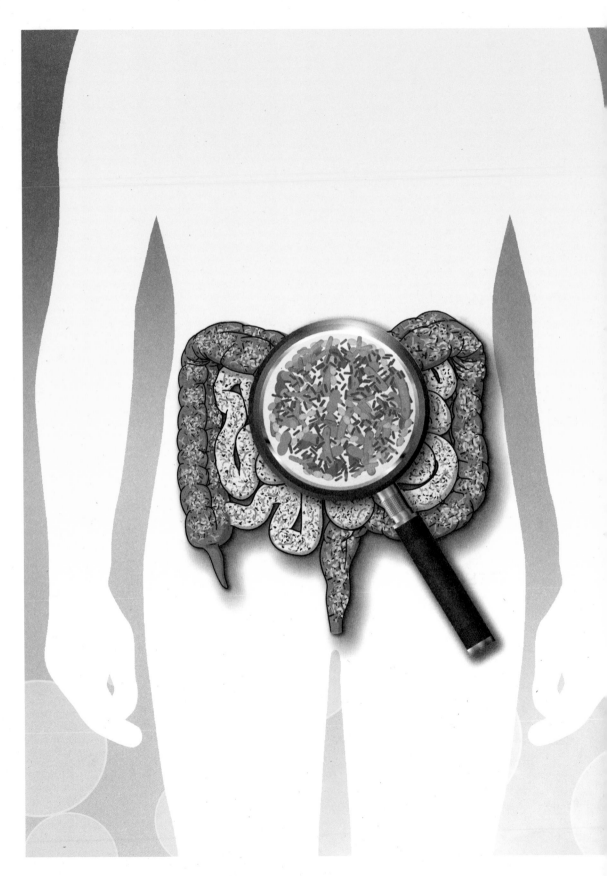

CHAPTER 1

A Great Extinction is Happening in YOUR GUT!

My point in this book is to share some new information you may never have heard before. There is a great extinction going on in your gut! What? Yes, that is correct, and it's called Loss of Microbial Diversity (LOMD).

So, what is microbial diversity, and why should I care if I'm losing it?

To best understand what microbial diversity means and why it is so essential to your health, please indulge me as I share a bit of basic information regarding the bacteria in your gut.

"Microbial diversity" refers to the over 1000 different species of tiny organisms that have been discovered living in and on our bodies. "Microbiome" is the collective name given to this collection of microbes, including bacteria, along with their DNA.

You house a literal ecosystem inside your digestive tract made up of 100 trillion microorganisms that outnumber - by ten times! - the individual cells that make up your entire body. Numerically speaking, you are only 10 percent human. The other 90 percent is primarily bacteria and other microbes such as yeasts, viruses, even parasites. It is no longer plausible to consider yourself as one being. You may now think of yourself in the plural, we rather than I.

"The microbiota is not accidental," says Dr. Martin Blaser, Director of the Center for Advanced Biotechnology and Medicine at Rutgers University and author of the book, *Missing Microbes*. "The microbiota has co-evolved with us over very long periods of time, and it performs beneficial functions for us, just as we perform beneficial functions for it...We are all working together as an ecological unit." [1]

THERE ARE 3 TYPES OF MICROBES IN THE GUT:

BENEFICIAL	COMMENSAL	PATHOGENIC
Large amount AKA probiotics	Small amount AKA neutral	Not found or very low levels AKA negative
Help maintain intestinal health	Neither beneficial or pathogenic	Present after contamination
Assist in digestion		Levels can increase as we age
Produce natural antibiotics		Cause dysbiosis and disease
Produce vitamins and enzymes		

An appropriate balance of those microbes, with beneficial bacteria far outweighing the others, makes the difference between the experience of vibrant health and unpleasant symptoms of chronic disease. The beneficial bacteria in your gut orchestrate numerous functions that will amaze you. I promise we will explore this fascinating community in more detail in future chapters.

By the way, examining bacterial diversity is a relatively recent focus of our scientific communities. People just weren't all that interested in studying poop!

Two groundbreaking studies are dramatically increasing awareness of the microbiome. The Human Microbiome Project[2] is a massive research initiative funded by the National Institutes of Health (NIH). It began in 2008 with the mission of identifying and characterizing the human microbiome. The project involved eighty universities and scientific institutions with an initial goal of defining the normal microbiome of healthy Westerners. It is also investigating how this great community of microbes is associated with human health and disease.

The American Gut and British Gut Projects are part of the Microsetta Initiative[3]. Scientists include citizen scientists (people in the general population) and academic and industry researchers. In other words, you, too, can contribute to this massive gut study!

I was a digestive care pioneer in my early clinics, personally assisting hundreds of people with their gut issues. Soon after that, I formulated unique nutritional supplementation to naturally help people in ways that weren't generally available on the consumer market. Working closely with professionals in the medical community, I was constantly researching the most up-to-the-minute breakthroughs relating to beneficial bacteria, known as probiotics.

The stool tests that I found valuable to help determine what was happening in the gut were in their infancy. As others in the integrative medical community realized the importance of understanding gut function, the testing improved and became more sensitive. I began to see glimpses of increased bacterial diversity as an excellent indicator of good health in those I supported clinically.

Check out these two real-life examples that led to my "aha!" moments concerning the power of microbial diversity:

In 2013, we used Genova Diagnostics' Comprehensive Stool Profile to gather the research behind my book, *The Skinny Gut Diet*. Our goal was to help individuals lose weight, increase energy, and improve mental clarity through dietary change and natural supplementation. We conducted multiple stool tests throughout our study and began to recognize an emerging pattern. Initial tests showed reduced beneficial bacteria, and in many cases, the presence of pathogenic organisms that indicate possible disease processes.

As participants lost weight and started feeling more robust and energetic, we observed a quantitative shift toward more beneficial bacteria, appropriate balance of the gut overall, and increased microbial diversity. Through diet and supplementation, microbial diversity was improving, and with that, weight loss, improved health, and feelings of well-being were the happy results. Not only did we have verbal testimonials and diminishing waistlines, but we could also see the results on paper in our follow-up testing!

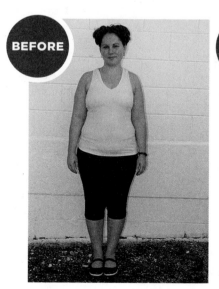 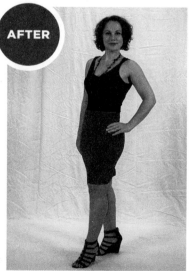

Danielle, a member of *The Skinny Gut Diet* project, lost 30 pounds!

In 2015, I participated in a clinical trial conducted through a northeastern hospital. We were interested in the impact of nutritional products on the health of seriously debilitated individuals who had survived colon cancer and other severe digestive disruptions. A part of the initial health screening we chose to do involved the type of testing I mentioned above. Genova's GI Effects offered next-generation testing protocols for gut study and had a pictorial representation (graphic below) to demonstrate the relative diversity of the patient's gut, "at-a-glance." As you might imagine, these people were almost without exception, showing dramatically "lower" diversity. The sicker a person was, the more barren and less diverse was their microbial gut environment. And these were some very ill people.

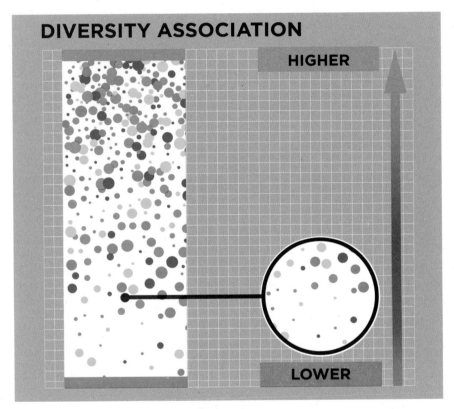

Let's get back to LOMD and why this understanding is so critical to your health. "LOMD" is the term used to describe this condition where we lose many of the different types of bacteria that should normally reside in our gut. Retaining diversity is desirable so the bacteria can work together harmoniously to keep us healthy.

Unfortunately, more and more people are suffering from LOMD and experiencing health challenges as a result. It has become the most common cause of gut bacterial imbalance.

It's possible that our future loved ones may be even MORE susceptible to chronic health issues than we are today.

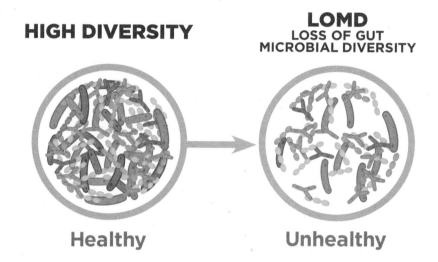

Let's delve into this new phenomenon by first taking a look back in time.

In the beginning, as a hunter-gatherer population, the human gut had a very high amount of microbial diversity. What that means is that previously we had a lot of different types (strains) of beneficial bacteria in our intestinal system.

As we progressed into a traditional farming and fishing population, we lost some strain diversity. But, overall, diversity remained relatively high.

However, as we progressed into an industrialized population, especially with the onset of processed foods, high sugar, and excessive carbohydrates, we started losing more and more of our beneficial bacterial strains.

GENERATIONAL - Loss of Microbial Diversity

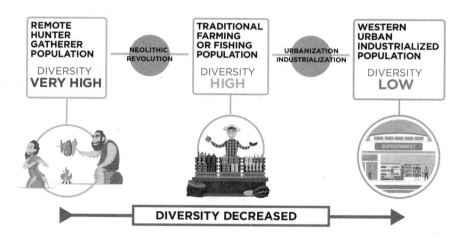

KEY POINT: Gradual loss of gut microbial diversity has occurred over generations due to changes in environment and diet. This loss has accelerated over the last 100 years.

Today, comparatively speaking, our microbial diversity is much lower in industrialized societies. It may be lower than it has ever been.

In addition, researchers believe that we will continue to lose essential strains of bacteria generation after generation. They've demonstrated this in a mouse study funded by NIH and conducted in 2016[4].

In this study, the investigators began with a wild field mouse that had eaten a natural wild diet.

In testing the bacterial content of the wild mouse stool, we see that the diversity of bacteria initially found was very high, as shown on the left side of this graph.

Generational Mouse Study
Showing Loss of Gut Bacterial Diversity

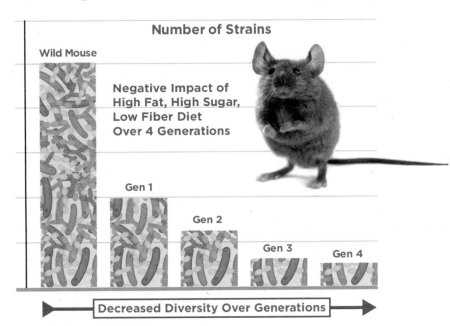

Sonnenburg, E., Smits, S., Tikhonov, M. *et al.* Diet-induced extinctions in the gut microbiota compound over generations. *Nature* **529**, 212–215 (2016).

Next, the investigators started feeding the mouse more processed foods high in fat and low in fiber, mimicking our Western diet. After breeding the mouse, they tested four generations of offspring.

This study was performed with mice because the generations manifest quickly.

The graph shows a decrease in the number of bacterial strains present with each successive generation. This study illustrates how microbial diversity drops dramatically by generation, especially compared to the original wild mouse. Bringing this research home, humans – such as you, your children, your grandchildren are also experiencing decreasing diversity through the generations.

Robust health is linked to a higher diversity of bacteria in our guts!

Other studies link a drop in microbial diversity in the gut to an increase in health issues. Have you noticed people facing challenges with chronic conditions like blood sugar issues, arthritis, cardiovascular issues, and obesity earlier in life?

Dan Knight, a well-known microbiologist, recently did a Ted Talk[5] highlighting a study he led using different monkey populations.

Knight's team observed that when these non-human primates transitioned from living in the wild into a zoo environment, they lost a significant amount of bacterial diversity. The change in diet from a "wild" setting to a more captive environment mirrors what has happened to humans throughout history. Our human microbial diversity has decreased as we have changed from a natural, plant-based diet to highly processed, sugary, and more fatty foods.

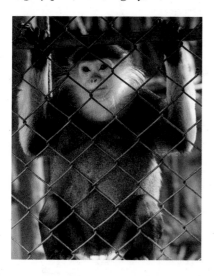

Sadly, the monkeys in captivity started demonstrating human-type diseases like obesity, gastroenteritis, diarrhea, and other health conditions which don't exist for primates in the wild.

As mentioned above, this is what seems to be happening generation after generation in the human population. If our behaviors continue down this current path, our grandchildren will likely have even fewer strains of beneficial bacteria in their guts than we have.

TO RECAP:

- There is a great extinction going on in your gut! It's called Loss of Microbial Diversity (LOMD).
- LOMD is the term used to describe the condition wherein we lose many different strains of bacteria that should normally reside in our gut and work together to keep us healthy.
- Researchers believe that we will continue to lose essential strains of bacteria generation after generation.
- Studies link a decrease in microbial diversity in the gut to an increase in chronic health issues such as digestive diseases, obesity, arthritis, cardiovascular problems, and more!

Top 10 causes of decreased gut diversity

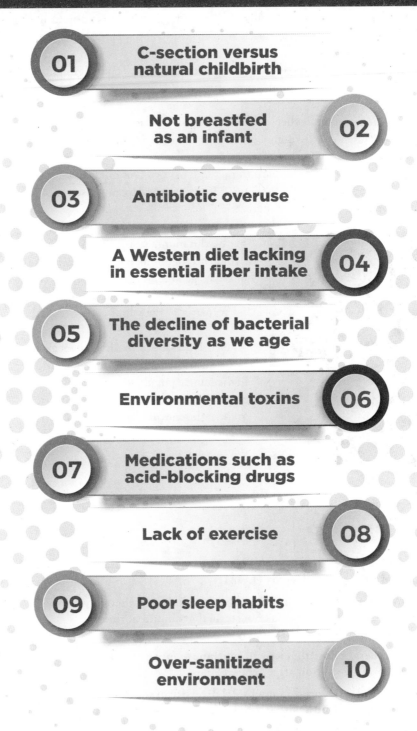

01 C-section versus natural childbirth

02 Not breastfed as an infant

03 Antibiotic overuse

04 A Western diet lacking in essential fiber intake

05 The decline of bacterial diversity as we age

06 Environmental toxins

07 Medications such as acid-blocking drugs

08 Lack of exercise

09 Poor sleep habits

10 Over-sanitized environment

CHAPTER 2

What Causes LOMD?

Now I hope you understand how LOMD has manifested, generationally and geographically. In this chapter, I would like to discuss contributing lifestyle factors increasing LOMD in our Western society. Awareness of these factors can go a long way toward supporting your microbial diversity - and improving it in many cases.

 C-section versus natural childbirth

One of the most significant benefits of natural childbirth is that the baby is exposed to many extremely beneficial bacterial strains as it passes through the birth canal.

This initial bath of good bacteria helps to establish the baby's "microbial footprint," which plays a highly supportive role in the baby's health as it grows. These early benefits may continue for their lifetime.[1]

Natural childbirth is very positive for the child, especially if the mother has a healthy environment of Lactobacillus and Bifidobacteria vaginally. This more diverse bacterial environment occurs when the mother maintains a healthy diet during pregnancy. A daily supplemental probiotic can also enhance the vaginal bacteria, assisting in establishing bacterial diversity in the developing baby.

With a C-section birth, the baby misses out on bathing in the vaginal microbiome completely. A C-section baby develops an entirely different microbial footprint than was naturally intended. Their bacterial footprint tends to be the bacteria found on the mother's skin and within the hospital environment.

Thank goodness that more and more doctors realize the importance of this initial exposure to mother's beneficial bacteria. In cases where a C-section is necessary, some doctors are now swabbing mother's vaginal cavity and wiping the bacteria onto the baby's skin after the procedure. Consider asking for this to be done if you are facing the potential of a C-section birth.

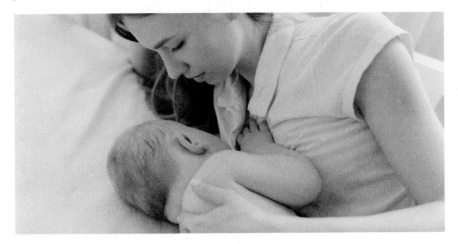

 Not breastfed as an infant

Another early childhood factor that helps determine microbial diversity is whether or not a child is breastfed.

Research has documented the many benefits of breastfeeding.[2,3] Concerning LOMD, beneficial bacteria are passed to the baby through the mother's breastmilk along with certain sugars that act as prebiotics. Some of the known benefits of breastfeeding to the infant throughout life are as follows:

- Lower risk of breast cancer
- Lower risk of ovarian cancer
- Lower risk of rheumatoid arthritis
- Less endometriosis
- Less osteoporosis with age
- Less diabetes
- Less hypertension; decreases blood pressure
- Less cardiovascular disease
- Lowers the risk of developing postpartum depression

Breastfeeding undoubtedly helps the baby establish bacterial diversity in the gut while supporting a healthy microbial footprint that may benefit them throughout their life.

Antibiotic overuse

The use of prescription antibiotics can have several adverse effects on gut bacteria and diversity.[4] We've known that antibiotics deplete the total number of beneficial bacteria found in the gut for a long time. The most disturbing realization is that they may wipe out an entire beneficial bacterial strain that would typically be part of your microbial footprint, sometimes for life. Antibiotics also alter metabolic activity and allow antibiotic-resistant organisms to take hold, leading to antibiotic-associated diarrhea and recurrent C-difficile infections. Disruption of gut bacteria can contribute to many of the common diseases that are rampant today.

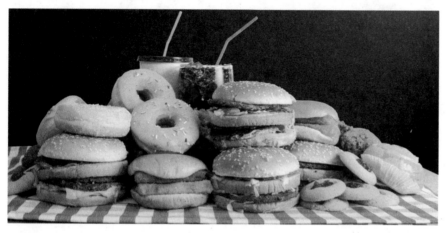

A Western diet lacking in essential fiber intake

I know you've heard this before! You can't ignore the negative impact the SAD (Standard American or Western Diet) has on our health overall. It's full of processed foods, high in sugar, and low in fiber. Excess sugars and carbohydrates often promote bacterial overgrowth, as harmful bacteria happily multiply on carbohydrates, resulting in digestive issues. Many times, the first noticed symptoms may be gas and bloating.

Concerning diversity, a high fiber diet provides prebiotics in that fiber itself is a prebiotic. As a result, fiber supplies food for a host of beneficial gut bacteria. Without food, probiotics can perish and certainly diminish in population.

What you eat (or don't eat) dramatically impacts your bacterial diversity, as is clearly shown by a 2017 study published by Stanford University Medical Center.[5] The focus of the study was the Hadza hunters in Tanzania, along with 17 other cultures around the world, some also hunter-gatherers.

This research found the Hadza's gut diversity was one of the richest on the planet. Their diet in the wet season consists almost entirely of food they forage from the forest, including wild berries, fiber-rich tubers, honey, and wild meat. They eat no processed food — or even food that comes from farms. Extremely high in various fibrous foods, their food is abundant in prebiotics which can support probiotics.

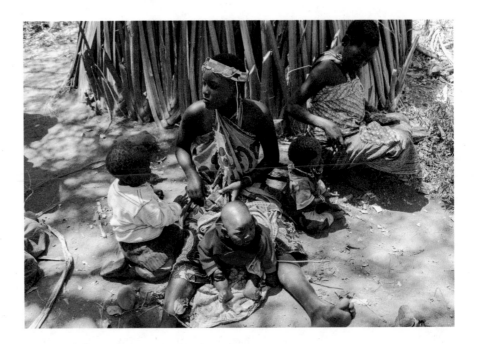

However, the Hadza's seasonal diet varies dramatically. This dietary alteration results in dramatic shifts in the diversity of their microbiota throughout the year. Interestingly, they eat much more meat in the dry season and less fresh food, including much less fiber. At the low point, their gut diversity drops and begins to resemble the guts found in our Western society.

Justin Sonnenburg, a microbiologist from Stanford U who has been studying the microbiome for ten years, states, "We're beginning to realize that people who eat more dietary fiber are actually feeding their gut microbiome."

The Hadza society consumes a massive amount of fiber because they eat fiber-rich tubers and fruit from baobab trees throughout much of the year. These staples give them about 100 to 150 grams of fiber each day in season. That's equivalent to the fiber in 50 bowls of Cheerios — and ten times more than many Americans eat. Take note - increasing fiber intake to at least 25-35 grams daily is a big step toward a healthier microbiome!

What exciting news! Perhaps, by shifting our Western diet, we may be able to reverse this great extinction in our guts over time!

> **"I think this finding (of the changing microbial composition) is really exciting," says Lawrence David, who studies the microbiome at Duke University. "It suggests the shifts in the microbiome seen in industrialized nations might not be permanent — that they might be reversible by changes in people's diets."** [6]

When it comes to bacterial diversity, fiber is your friend for three main reasons:

- **It stimulates bowel movements.**
- **It slows the absorption of sugar from other foods.**
- **Most importantly, regarding diversity, it acts as food for your beneficial gut bacteria.**

Bottom line, the foods you choose daily offer your body the building blocks required for healthy function. Proper digestion of your choices can then build a healthy gut. They are also absorbed into the bloodstream as nutrients to sustain strength and vitality.

You may have heard the phrase, "You are what you eat." Even more correctly, "you are what you absorb."

A diversity of probiotics is essential to this process. And probiotics depend on your food choices to survive and thrive!

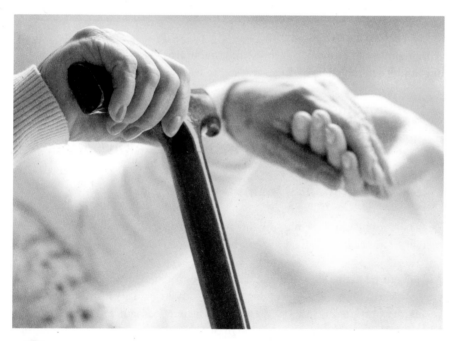

 The decline of bacterial diversity as we age

Next on our list is aging. As the years pass, there comes a decline in so many areas of life - energy levels, mental vigor, libido - and gut bacteria![7] As overall bacterial diversity decreases, the levels of your critical Bifidobacteria are hit hardest with age. Bifidobacteria comprise the majority of beneficial bacteria in the gut and reside primarily in the large intestine. Bifido produces acetic and lactic acids, substances that directly inhibit pathogenic bacteria.

Additionally, Bifidobacteria produce B vitamins, such as folic acid, and help absorb nutrients. They also have an integral role in producing short-chain fatty acids that feed the colon's lining, fortifying that essential barrier. LOMD concerning Bifidobacteria is an often-overlooked factor in the unpleasant stresses of aging.

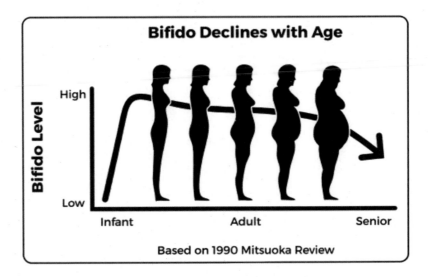

Bifido Declines with Age

Based on 1990 Mitsuoka Review

Although we can't do much to stop the aging process, we CAN help re-establish our bifidobacteria balance. Keep reading to learn more!

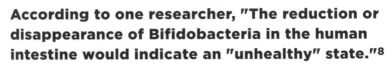

According to one researcher, "The reduction or disappearance of Bifidobacteria in the human intestine would indicate an "unhealthy" state."[8]

 Environmental toxins

Let's talk now about the environment. Toxins such as chlorine, fluoride, lead, and mercury can negatively affect our gut bacteria.[9]

Manufactured toxins are everywhere in our lives today. Sadly, they are in the very air we breathe. Some of the most dangerous toxins are actually inside of our house versus the outside air. Processed foods and drinks contain a plethora of toxic additives. We also absorb toxins through our skin via personal care products like make-up and shampoos. These manmade chemicals disrupt the beneficial bacterial balance in our gut microbiome. Exposure to these chemicals daily negatively impacts diversity by:

- Killing off beneficial bacterial strains
- Upsetting the natural way microbes multiply
- Disturbing nutrient absorption resulting in malabsorption
- Creating hormone imbalances - ex: estrogen

Fibrous foods and beneficial bacteria help process and eliminate toxins through your bowel movement.

> **Research shows that postnatal exposure of the baby to chemicals like in personal care products decreases diversity later in life.**[10]

It is a challenge to navigate our toxic environment. Education is key. The Environmental Working Group (EWG) has excellent information on what foods are toxic and heavily sprayed. They also offer consumer guides to skin products and sunscreen, household cleaners, water quality, and much more. Check them out at https://www.ewg.org/

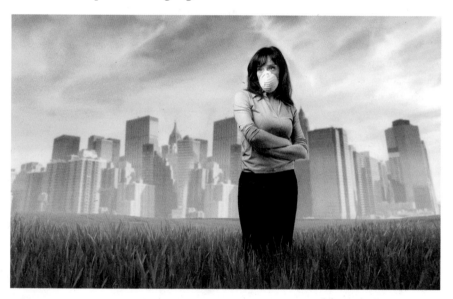

 Medications such as acid-blocking drugs

Besides antibiotics, many drugs can disrupt your gut bacteria. Acid-blocking medications are some of the worst culprits in our society, leading to LOMD.[11]

Why are they so harmful? We need our stomach acid! It helps control pathogenic bacteria from getting into the intestines. We also need it to regulate proper pH so our beneficial bacteria can thrive. Hydrochloric acid is one of nature's most essential pathogenic microbe killers. It helps destroy pathogens entering from the outside world, thus warding off disease.

There are two groups of acid-blocking drugs: H2 receptor blockers and proton pump inhibitors (PPIs).

H2 blockers prevent acid secretion by blocking the action of histamine. Histamine signals acid-blocking cells to secrete HCl upon command of the hormone gastrin. These drugs were originally developed to treat peptic ulcers. When medical professionals realized that ulcers were caused by H. pylori infection and not excess HCl, doctors used these drugs to treat gastroesophageal reflux disease (GERD). Sadly for the patients, H2 blockers cut off the production of stomach acid for hours at a time and, as a result, have serious side effects including GI disturbances such as:

- Constipation
- Diarrhea
- Nausea
- Vomiting
- B12 deficiency
- Dementia
- Heart attack
- Heartburn (the very reason you are taking them in the first place!)

Proton Pump Inhibitors (PPIs) reduce the experience of heartburn by inhibiting specific stomach cells from "pumping" acid into the stomach. They are the most potent form of acid-blocking medication. Buyer beware! - Long term use of PPI's is associated with increased risk of serious health issues such as:

- Pneumonia
- C-difficile infections
- Osteoporosis-related bone fracture
- Nutrient malabsorption, and more...

Acid-blocking medication quickly leads to dependency and attempts to stop their use can be extremely difficult. A "rebound effect" commonly occurs, causing worse symptoms than when the drug was initiated.

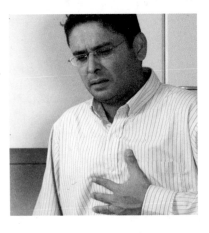

Harmful bacteria not destroyed in the stomach can proliferate and change the pH of the digestive tract. This environment sets up the digestive tract for an overgrowth of fungus and yeast. Long-term use has commonly been linked to conditions like IBS and SIBO, to name a couple.

Logically, you might think the reason to take acid-blocking meds is that you have too much acid in your stomach. Sadly, and often, the person with the burning in their gut has too little acid production, which in itself is a health concern. Using acid blockers only compounds this issue. The symptoms in both situations are almost identical! It's only recently that professionals understand this critical fact.

Unfortunately, acid-blocking medications were approved to be sold over-the-counter, without a prescription. Now anyone can take as much and for as long as they want, ignorant of the underlying side effects.

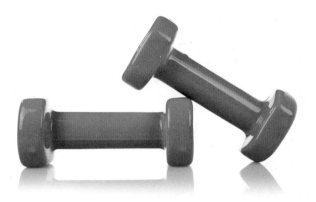

 08 **Lack of exercise**

And then let's consider possible lifestyle choices - like lack of exercise aka ("I'll start tomorrow...".)

It is no surprise that exercise stimulates the function of many muscles in the body, depending on what activity you choose. Although not the kind of muscle that you usually think of working out at the gym, your intestinal tract is also a muscle that is stimulated by movement.

Exercise can stimulate your nervous system and lower stress responses associated with "fight-or-flight" mechanisms, allowing you to de-stress, supporting good digestion.

Problems with elimination and impaired function of the nervous system set the perfect stage for LOMD. The vagus nerve specifically along with your enteric nervous system which is embedded in your intestine work together to help you produce a healthy bowel movement. This will be discussed further in Chapter 3.

Recent research has shown that exercise can increase microbial diversity, independent of diet. Participants in one study followed a 3-times weekly exercise program for six weeks.[12] They then reverted to a sedentary lifestyle for six weeks. With the help of fecal samples and genetic testing, the researchers found that all participants experienced an increase in SCFAs (short-chain fatty acid levels), which are a medically recognized positive indicator of colon health. They also discovered a rise in levels of various beneficial gut microbes that produce SCFAs following the exercise program. In other words, exercise helped create more and different good bacteria. However, these levels declined when subjects reverted to sedentary behavior.

A scientific review article published in 2016 summarized the findings of many different exercise-based studies. It explains how "Exercise Modifies the Gut Microbiota with Positive Health Effects."[13] The conclusion states that "Exercise is able to enrich the microflora diversity." (and the article continues...). I find that very encouraging!

09 Poor sleep habits

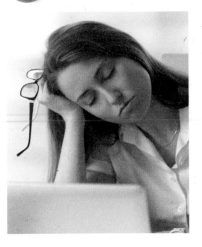

Poor sleep can increase stress in several ways, which can affect your microbial diversity.

As cortisol, the stress hormone rises, along with disrupted vagus nerve function, efficient movement of matter through the intestine is impaired. This dysfunction leads to a toxic gut environment decreasing microbial diversity and stimulating chronic inflammation throughout the body. Constipation, diarrhea, gas, and bloating are a few of the potential side effects.

The connection between sleep and appetite is well documented. Lack of sleep decreases the level of the hormone leptin, which is in charge of our hunger. Daily food choices directly affect microbial diversity, and hunger levels can lead to poor food decisions, encouraging LOMD.

Poor sleep due to lack of the sleep hormone melatonin may be related to the digestive condition known as gastroesophageal reflux disease (GERD). GERD is another sign of LOMD.

Conversely, gut bacteria influence normal sleep patterns by helping to create important chemical relaxation messengers in the brain like serotonin and dopamine. Research has revealed that both lack of bacterial diversity and microbe depletion negatively impact serotonin in the gut, thus affecting our body's natural rhythms and potentially disturbing sleep.[14]

Have symptoms of heartburn or possible gas and bloating ever disrupted your rest? These are some of the first signs of loss of microbial diversity, often initiated by going to sleep on a full stomach.

We will discuss these processes in more detail in subsequent chapters.

Ultimately, since the gut-brain connection works both ways, If you're getting insufficient sleep, it certainly makes sense that it would negatively impact gut health.

TIP

Allow 3 hours after your last meal before laying down to sleep to support proper digestion.

Over-sanitized environment

And finally, let's address our over-sanitized environment. Science shows us that exposure to a variety of microbes contributes to the diversity of our microbial footprint, thus strengthening our immune systems, beginning in childhood. Studies on children raised with animals have demonstrated a more resilient immune system than children who are not. So yes, let the dog lick the baby or let the baby lick the dog! [15]

Recent studies are exploring the effects of antibacterial cleaning products on the human microbiome. Antibacterial and antibiotic are synonyms. We previously discussed the complications associated with antibiotic overuse.

Seasonal colds and flu stimulate practical recommendations to wash our hands frequently and clean surfaces diligently. However, overzealous habitual disinfecting of ourselves and our habitats can alter our natural environment's microbial diversity and inadvertently lead to the creation of antibiotic-resistant genes, both externally and internally. [16]

There are many ways we can lose our microbial diversity, too many times resulting in chronic health issues.

Ultimately, it all comes full circle, right back to listening to your gut - the core to your health.

TO RECAP:

Many lifestyle factors can contribute to the development of LOMD. These can include:

- C-section versus natural childbirth
- Not breastfed as an infant
- Antibiotic overuse
- A Western diet lacking in essential fiber intake
- The decline of bacterial diversity as we age
- Environmental toxins
- Medications such as acid-blocking drugs
- Lack of exercise
- Poor sleep habits
- Over-sanitized environment

Awareness of these factors can go a long way toward supporting your microbial diversity - and improving your health in many cases.

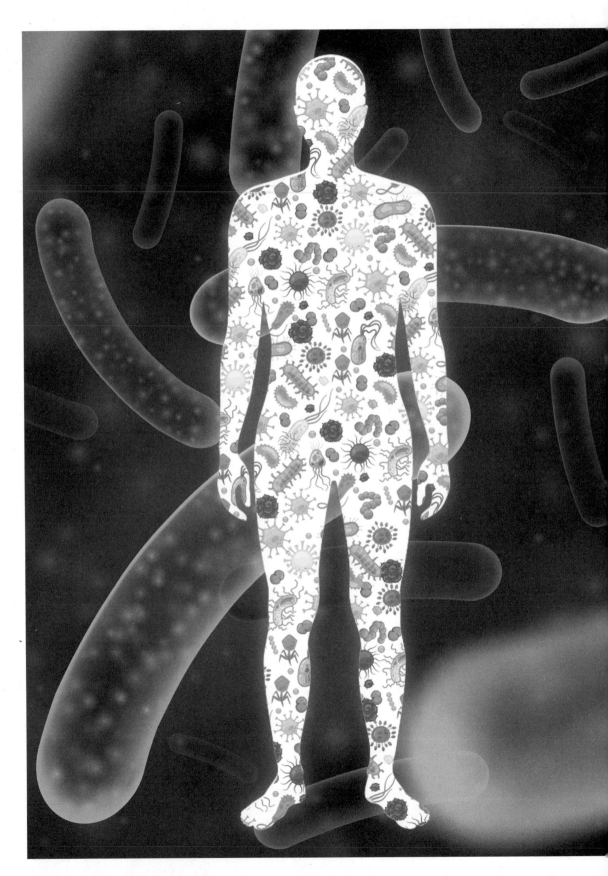

CHAPTER 3

DIVERSITY and the MICROBIOME

Probiotics are a popular subject, and all the noise
can sometimes be confusing.

I'd like to offer you a deeper understanding of probiotics and why diversity is
so important.

Let's start with the basics. The word PROBIOTIC literally means FOR LIFE.
We define them as organisms living inside and on us that have a beneficial function
for the health of the human body.

The microbiome is not only living bacteria but also includes some helpful types
of yeast and other micro-organisms. In our discussions, I may also refer to them
as "beneficial microflora" or "good microbes."

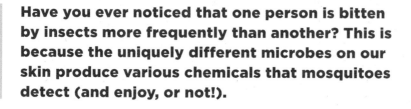

**Have you ever noticed that one person is bitten
by insects more frequently than another? This is
because the uniquely different microbes on our
skin produce various chemicals that mosquitoes
detect (and enjoy, or not!).**

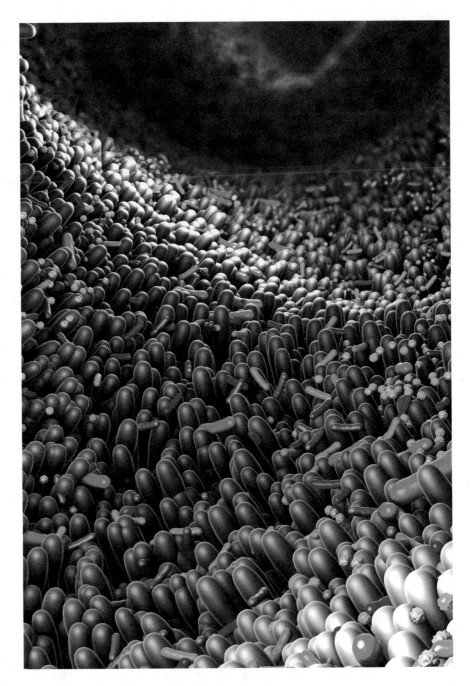

Rob Knight, the lead researcher in the Human Microbiome Project funded by the NIH, divides bacterial communities into four areas - skin, oral, vaginal, and intestinal, with the overwhelming majority of the microflora residing in the gut. All these microbes are collectively referred to as the "microbiome."[1]

As a reminder, we have 100 trillion bacterial cells within the gut, with the small intestine home to a few billion and the large intestine supporting 10s of trillions. This bacterial population amounts to approximately 3 to 4 pounds, roughly the weight of a brick. In fact, bacteria make up 60-80 percent of the dry mass of your stool.

8 PRIMARY PURPOSES OF PROBIOTICS

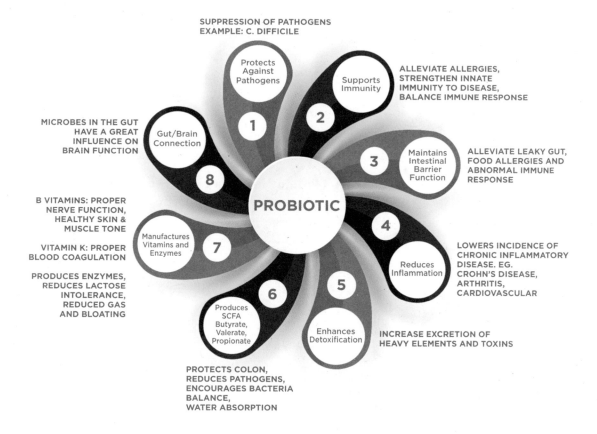

SUPPRESSION OF PATHOGENS
EXAMPLE: C. DIFFICILE

ALLEVIATE ALLERGIES, STRENGTHEN INNATE IMMUNITY TO DISEASE, BALANCE IMMUNE RESPONSE

MICROBES IN THE GUT HAVE A GREAT INFLUENCE ON BRAIN FUNCTION

ALLEVIATE LEAKY GUT, FOOD ALLERGIES AND ABNORMAL IMMUNE RESPONSE

B VITAMINS: PROPER NERVE FUNCTION, HEALTHY SKIN & MUSCLE TONE

VITAMIN K: PROPER BLOOD COAGULATION

PRODUCES ENZYMES, REDUCES LACTOSE INTOLERANCE, REDUCED GAS AND BLOATING

LOWERS INCIDENCE OF CHRONIC INFLAMMATORY DISEASE. EG. CROHN'S DISEASE, ARTHRITIS, CARDIOVASCULAR

INCREASE EXCRETION OF HEAVY ELEMENTS AND TOXINS

PROTECTS COLON, REDUCES PATHOGENS, ENCOURAGES BACTERIA BALANCE, WATER ABSORPTION

1 Protects Against Pathogens
2 Supports Immunity
3 Maintains Intestinal Barrier Function
4 Reduces Inflammation
5 Enhances Detoxification
6 Produces SCFA Butyrate, Valerate, Propionate
7 Manufactures Vitamins and Enzymes
8 Gut/Brain Connection

PROBIOTIC

Most people think that probiotics are only valuable for gut health and immunity. They don't realize the wide range of other health benefits they offer.

It's amazing to think that most health problems can be traced back to an imbalance of gut microflora, some more directly than others of course. As an expert in probiotics, I've developed a list of the eight primary roles of probiotics.

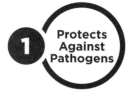

The first role probiotics play in our health is protection against pathogenic organisms and infections.

As an example, consider a few disease-related organisms like certain types of E. coli or Clostridia difficile.

These harmful organisms can quickly take over the intestinal system and lead to dangerous, even deadly infections. Our good MICROFLORA helps this from happening in two ways.

Probiotics compete for space in the gut with pathogenic organisms. They also fight for food sources that help them both thrive.

The more beneficial microflora we have in our gut, the less space and food available for pathogenic bacteria to increase. As you now realize, too many harmful bacteria can lead to serious health problems.

Good bacteria also produce a byproduct called lactic acid. Our microflora thrives in this acidic environment, but pathogenic organisms do not. A high amount of probiotics in our gut naturally creates an unfriendly environment for negative bacteria.

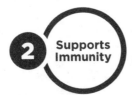

2 **Supports Immunity** **Probiotics play a critical supportive role in the development of both our innate and acquired immune systems.**

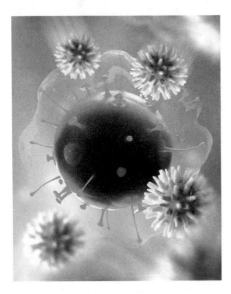

Your innate immune system gets its name because we are born with some factors in place that continue development shortly after birth. Your acquired immune system develops and changes over the course of your lifetime and learns from every exposure to a new substance.

Exposure to the maternal bacteria during birth and breast feeding initiates the development of the immune cells within the innate immune system. The bacteria teach these immune cells how to respond to unknown invaders.

Probiotics also stimulate production of an antibody in the small intestine called secretory IGA. Secretory IGA is the first line of defense against viruses, pathogenic bacteria and parasites and is part of your acquired immune system.

Our beneficial bacteria in the gut also communicate to other organs around the body such as the liver, the brain and the lungs and helps teach them how to develop appropriate immune cells.

It is our bacteria that keeps our immune systems strong and responding appropriately.

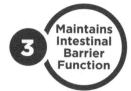

3 Maintains Intestinal Barrier Function

Probiotics help maintain the function of our intestinal barrier. Most likely, you've heard about the condition called "Leaky Gut." The medical term for this condition is "Increased Intestinal Permeability."

It's commonly known as leaky gut because when the intestinal lining becomes permeable, it allows harmful organisms to pass through the gut lining and enter the bloodstream. Not a good thing.

Probiotics help maintain the integrity of our intestinal lining, so this doesn't occur.

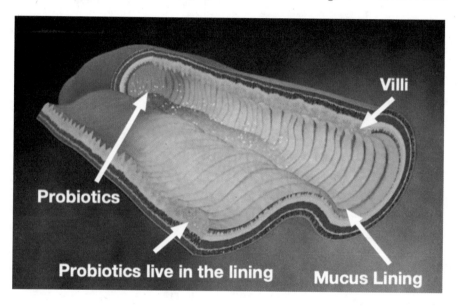

Villi

Probiotics

Probiotics live in the lining

Mucus Lining

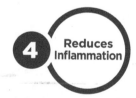

4 Reduces Inflammation

Probiotics help reduce the development of chronic inflammation in the body.

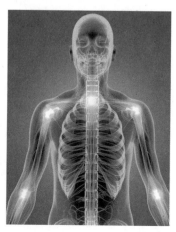

We know that ongoing, chronic inflammation is very damaging to the body, especially the cardiovascular system.

Probiotics increase the production of the anti-inflammatory proteins in our bodies called "cytokines." These types of cytokines ensure a healthier inflammatory response.

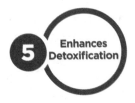

Probiotics help to enhance our body's natural detoxification process.

For example, some probiotics can bind with heavy metals in the gut. These include mercury, lead, cadmium, and arsenic. Once bound, the body can then excrete them in the bowel movement. (Remember that the bowel movement is 60-80 percent bacteria.)

Probiotics can also help break down environmental pesticide residues on our food that end up in our bodies. One example is glyphosate.

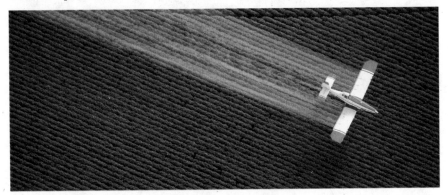

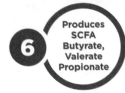

Probiotics produce short-chain fatty acids (SCFA) within the colon. These include butyrate, valerate, and proprionate. These are made when the bacteria in our gut ferment the fiber in our diet.

Short-chain fatty acids are critical to the health of our colon cells. They act as food for the cells, stimulating colon cell growth.

A shortage of probiotics may mean less short-chain fatty acids and less turnover of our colon cells, leading to increased inflammation! Therefore, to ensure a healthy colon, we require those colon cells to reproduce. In fact, most GI doctors measure butyrate levels to help determine the health of the colon.

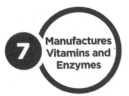

Probiotics support the digestion of our nutrients and manufacture vitamins. Our gut bacteria have the ability to produce digestive enzymes.

Enzymes are vitally important because they assist in the breakdown of our food (known as digestion). Probiotics may produce protease, amylase, and lipase, which digest protein, carbohydrates, and fats.

Our food must be thoroughly broken down to absorb nutrients efficiently. Additionally, fully digested food reduces fermentation, which creates gas and bloating. Probiotics also play a role in reducing the symptoms of lactose intolerance (problems digesting dairy).

Our microflora also helps to manufacture essential vitamins - B vitamins & vitamin K.

The many notable roles of B vitamins have been appreciated for a long time - proper nerve function, healthier skin and muscle tone, along with my favorite, regularity, to name a few. We are just starting to appreciate the valuable benefits of vitamin K. First and foremost, vitamin K is essential for proper blood clotting.

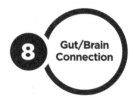

Microbes in the gut have a significant influence on brain function. It's time to peek at the fantastic Gut-Brain Connection!

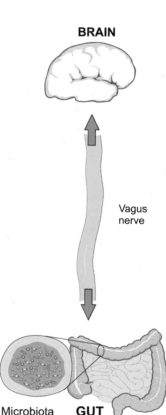

1. A healthy and diverse microbiome is critical to the gut-brain connection by supporting healthy digestive function. In addition, probiotics and their byproducts offer many benefits to the brain, including:

• Decrease inflammation in the brain by way of strengthening the blood-brain barrier

• Improves mood and reduces anxiety

• Communicate with the vagus nerve

• Help with the production of brain neurotransmitters, like serotonin and GABA

2. The vagus nerve is the main component of the parasympathetic nervous system, which carries a significant range of signals from the microbes of the digestive system and organs to the brain and vice versa.

• The vagus nerve controls peristalsis, regulates the production of stomach acid, and supports many other digestive processes.

• Having sub-optimal vagus nerve function can increase the chances of developing digestive issues.

HOW ARE PROBIOTICS NAMED?

Bear with me here. This information will be very important shortly.

Probiotics have three names, just like people. First, middle, and last. The only way to identify a specific probiotic is by knowing all three names.
First = genus
Middle = species
Last = strain
For example - Lactobacillus acidophilus VPLA-4

It is important to know all 3 names because probiotic functions vary at the *strain level* although they all work together as a team. For example, one strain of acidophilus may be better at supporting immunity, whereas another strain might be more effective at reducing inflammation. It is the effect of all of them combined that gives us the most supportive health benefits overall.

This is not an exact science at this point in time, as we are still in the discovery phase of these dynamic interactions.

Each strain provides its own health benefits

STRAIN	SUPPORTS IMMUNITY	REDUCES INFLAMMATION	MAKES VITAMINS	PROTECTS AGAINST PATHOGENS
L.acidophilus VPLA-4	GREAT	GREAT	GOOD	BEST
L.acidophilus NCFM	FAIR	BEST	GREAT	GOOD
L.acidophilus VP-35	BEST	GOOD	FAIR	GREAT
L.acidophilus HA-122	GREAT	GREAT	BEST	FAIR

This chart is only an example of the diversity concept I have described.

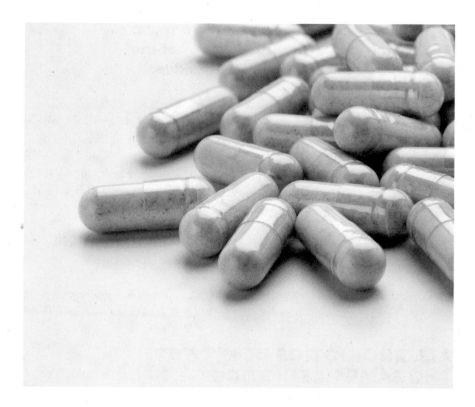

In the 25 years I've been working with probiotic formulas, research and understanding have advanced tremendously.

WHAT WE USED TO THINK WAS TRUE...
THAT WE NOW KNOW IS WRONG.

- There were only hundreds of strains in our gut.
- There was only one strain of each species (i.e., acidophilus) in our gut.
- All strains of each species were the same genetically.
- All strains of each species provided the same set of health benefits.
- All we needed was a single strain of each species for optimal health.

WHAT WE NOW KNOW TO BE TRUE.

- We have *thousands* of strains in our gut, not hundreds.
- There are *many strains of the same species* (i.e., acidophilus) in our gut, not just one.
- Each species has *many genetically different strains* (for example, there are 250+ L. acidophilus strains, each with a unique genetic footprint.)
- Each genetically different strain *provides its own specific set of health benefits.*
- We *need multiple strains of each species* to achieve and maintain optimal health.

We now know that probiotic formulas should include multiple strains of the same species to be most effective.

A fundamental note! Beneficial bacteria thrive on certain soluble fibers from the foods we eat. They are known as prebiotics because they act as food for probiotics. A diet that includes prebiotics is essential for a healthy microbiome. I'm sure you remember the Hadza hunter-gatherers from Chapter 2 and the exceptional bacterial diversity they demonstrated in their guts during times when they were eating copious amounts of fibrous foods. We will discuss the value of dietary fiber much more in upcoming chapters.

As I embraced these cutting-edge realizations, I began to recognize that the key to a healthy microbiome, as well as a healthy world, is DIVERSITY!

Like in the rainforest, where biodiversity is high, a diverse variety of organisms in your gut helps maintain the health of the ecosystem - which in this case is YOU!

ALL PROBIOTICS DON'T EAT THE SAME PREBIOTICS

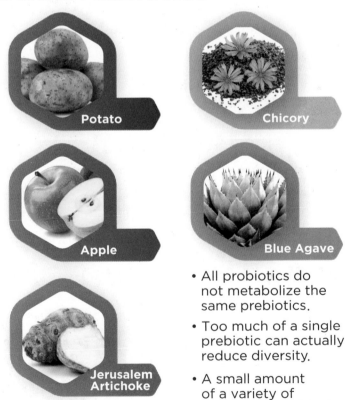

Potato

Chicory

Apple

Blue Agave

Jerusalem Artichoke

- All probiotics do not metabolize the same prebiotics.
- Too much of a single prebiotic can actually reduce diversity.
- A small amount of a variety of prebiotics is critical.

KEY POINT: Multi-strain probiotic formulas need multiple prebiotics.

TO RECAP:

- Probiotics are organisms living inside of us, and on us, that provide beneficial functions for our health.
- There are three types of organisms (microbes) in the gut - beneficial, commensal, and pathogenic.
- An imbalance of your microbial community may lead to various issues and, ultimately, disease processes.

The 8 primary roles that probiotics within microflora play in our health:

1. They help protect us against pathogenic organisms and infections.
2. They support our immune system.
3. Probiotics help maintain the integrity of our intestinal lining.
4. They support a healthy inflammatory response.
5. Probiotics enhance our body's detoxification processes.
6. They produce short-chain fatty acids which support colon health.
7. They support the digestion of nutrients and manufacture vitamins B & K.
8. Probiotics strongly influence brain function.

- Probiotics have three names - genus, species, and strain.
- Probiotic functions vary at the strain level.
- There are thousands of strains of bacteria in our microbiome.
- We need multiple strains of each species for vibrant health.

So here's one more very important fact that I want to leave you with today:

Some - not all - bacteria strains work better at each of these eight functions than others.

Having the appropriate strains to perform key roles in the body is why high strain diversity is critical. The more probiotic strains we have, the more we can support these necessary functions that keep us healthy.

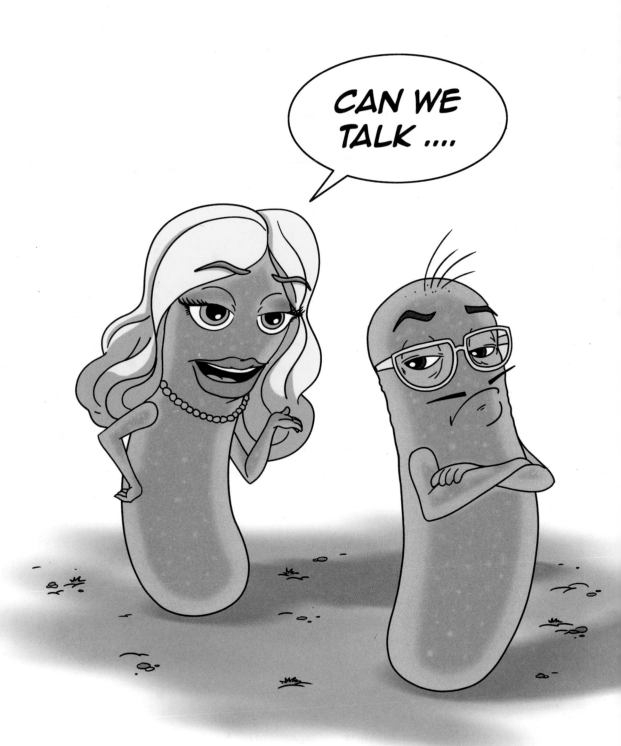

CHAPTER 4

CAN WE TALK?
QUORUM SENSING
AND THE GUT

This chapter is so exciting for me. Many years ago, I lectured around the country on how probiotics benefit human health. At that time, most people considered bacteria "the enemy," and the only proper way to deal with them was with a can of Lysol or chlorine bleach!

I often presented with a medical doctor by the name of Dr. Leonard Smith. He was a brilliant surgeon and well-known expert on gut health. We were teaching digestive wellness long before the NIH funded the Microbiome Project in 2008, which we mentioned in Chapter 1. The research projects that have continued since that time have completely transformed scientific awareness regarding bacteria in the gut.

Dr. Smith and I had a favorite presentation we called "The Lost Organ: Gut Bacteria." He believed that gut bacteria communicated among themselves and used to explain that our gut bacteria are like a symphony with a conductor. The conductor is the communicator between all the different musical instruments and the people playing them. His analogy was that our gut bacteria operated similarly. The bacteria had a communicator that kept all the beneficial, commensal, and pathogenic bacteria in sync so that they could make lovely music together. I was always amazed by Dr. Smith's insights. Over time the scientific understandings of the microbiome revealed that Dr. Smith was right on target.

We now know that our bacteria communicate with each other through a process called quorum sensing (QS). It is a cell-to-cell communication that allows bacteria to share information. QS was first discovered in the mid-1960s by Hungarian microbiologist Alexander Tomasz in his research on Streptococcus pneumonia. However, a microbiologist by the name of Dr. Bonnie Bassler has significantly expanded on this particular research. She recently did a Ted Talk explaining some of her team's fascinating discoveries. I strongly suggest you take 15 minutes to listen to her presentation.[1]

Her team's research involved a particular marine bacteria species called Vibrio fischeri. This species of bacteria lives in a little squid off the coast of Hawaii called the Hawaiian Bobtail Squid. These squids exude bioluminescence at night, meaning they glow. Dr. Bassler's team discovered that the glow was due to Vibrio fischeri and not the actual squid. The bacteria themselves absorb light during the day and glow at night. Although this in itself is fascinating, what is even more intriguing is that when her team isolated the bacteria, diluted them, and looked at just one organism – it would not produce light. However, when the bacteria were grouped back together, light was created. And all the bacteria turned on their lights in unison!

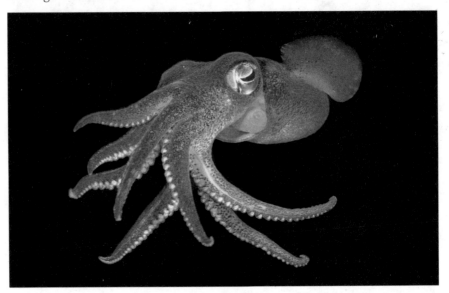

Next, the question was posed "How did the bacteria know when they were alone or in community with other bacteria?" The researchers discovered that Vibrio fischeri talked to each via a chemical language. The bacteria knew when they were together and had reached a large enough majority (hence a quorum) to act as a group. With that information, the research team then looked at how this may play a role in the human body and the bacteria that inhabit us.

Technical definition of quorum - the minimum number of members of an assembly or society that must be present at any of its meetings to make the proceedings of that meeting valid.[2]

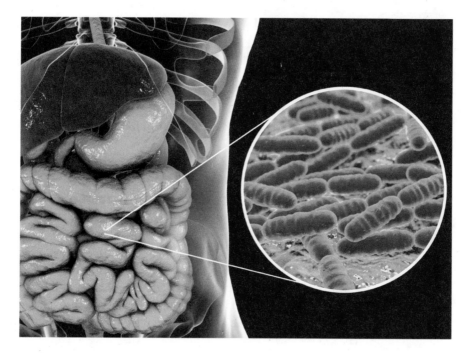

As you know, bacteria are single-celled organisms and extremely tiny, microscopic in fact. You have learned as well, regarding human health, that there are both beneficial and harmful bacteria. Have you ever wondered how such a tiny organism can do anything good, or for that matter anything bad, for us or to us?

Well, they can't – not by themselves anyway. This is where quorum sensing comes into play within the human body. Dr. Bassler and her team discovered that it takes the bacteria communicating with one another and joining together as a group for them to provide a benefit or cause disease.

To explain further, Dr. Bassler has discovered that both good and bad bacteria excrete a chemical messenger (similar to a hormone) called an autoinducer. Each species of bacteria excrete specific autoinducers so they can communicate with their own kind. Interestingly, they also secret another autoinducer that enables them to communicate among different species. Imagine if there was a universal human language that we all recognized that allowed us to communicate with anyone worldwide. That would be pretty amazing, don't you think?

This exact communication process happens among bacteria and is involved in many, if not all, aspects of what our gut bacteria do. QS allows our bacteria to recognize how many of themselves are present, how many other species are present, and who is declining or increasing in number.

With greater diversity of bacteria come more of these chemical messengers (autoinducers), resulting in better communication among our bacterial community. Conversely, the lower our diversity and population of bacteria get, the weaker communication becomes. Once a bacterial quorum is reached, the specific activity of that species can commence. In the case of Vibrio fischeri, everyone glows!

I'm sure you can now see how effective communication enhances the abilities of our gut bacteria to perform their many vital functions. The clearer the messaging, the better our gut bacteria can fulfill all their many critical functions. These include but are not limited to the 8 Primary Purposes outlined in the last chapter. Additionally, our gut bacteria communicate with each other regarding their immediate environment and respond accordingly to the betterment of their group. Bacteria are continually adjusting to changes in our food, toxins, and stress levels, for example.[3]

Technical definition of quorum sensing (QS) - the regulation of gene expression in response to fluctuations in cell-population density.[4]

It's important to note that beneficial bacteria are not the only ones that communicate. Pathogenic organisms do as well. One single pathogenic organism will not cause you damage by itself. Through the production of chemical messengers, the pathogens sense how many of their kind are present. Concurrently, the bacteria evaluate the environment, including the number of good bacteria that present potential interference to their activity. In a conducive setting, once a quorum is reached, the pathogens will then, in unison, execute the appropriate action for the species, possibly harming the host in the process. Hopefully, the host is not you. This process is called the virulence factor, or rather the ability of an organism to cause disease. With bacteria, it depends on QS communication.[5]

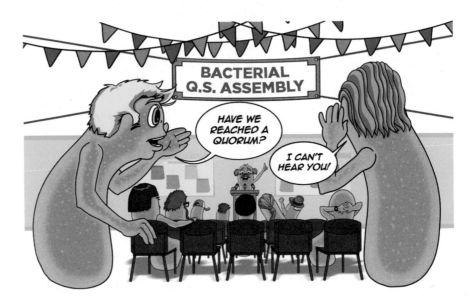

Quorum sensing is also involved in the formation of bacterial biofilms, a type of protective shell that some pathogenic bacteria create. An example of biofilm formation was first described in the 17th century when Anton Von Leeuwenhoek - the inventor of the microscope, saw microbial aggregates (now known to be biofilms) on scraping plaque from his teeth.

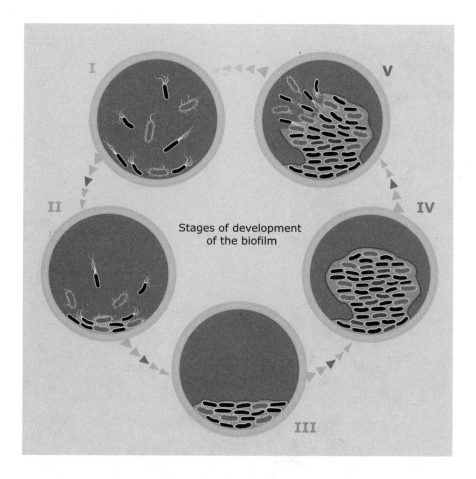

Stages of development
of the biofilm

The term "biofilm" was coined in 1978. Since then, research has repeatedly demonstrated that biofilms are prevalent in dysbiosis and disease. Biofilms can shield pathogens from medication designed to destroy them.

Bacteria growing in a biofilm are highly resistant to antibiotics, 1,000 to 1,500 times more resistant than the same bacteria not growing in a biofilm.[6]

A deeper understanding of how bacteria communicate will undoubtedly prove extremely helpful in deterring pathogenic infections or, conversely, encourage the effects of our good bacterial communities. Imagine if we could interrupt the communication of harmful bacteria not to organize an "attack"! Or if we might enhance chemical messengers to direct the beneficial bacteria on what to do and when to promote health!

Microbial communication is an emerging science that is awe-inspiring and exciting. I just wish Leonard was still here to see it all happen.

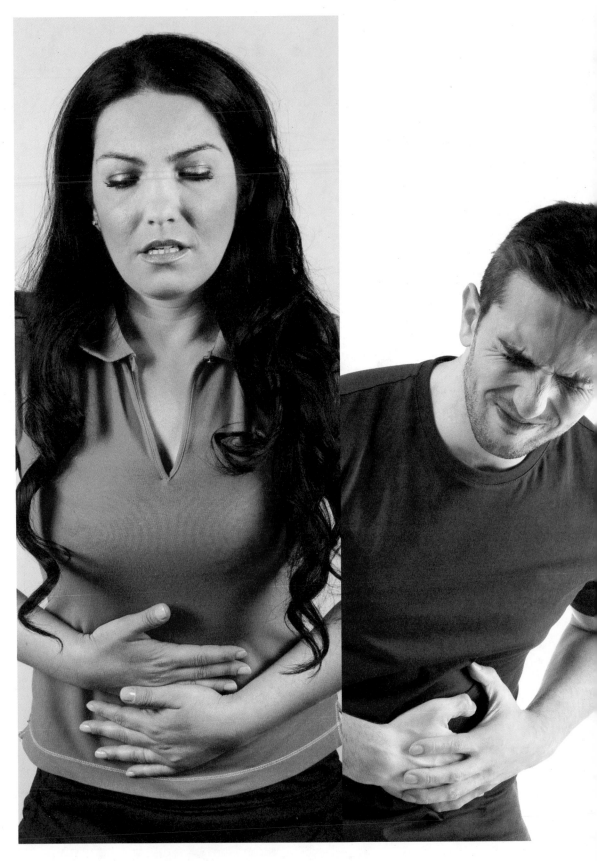

CHAPTER 5

FIRST SIGNS of LOMD

Perhaps as you read through the previous chapters, you noticed that I mentioned various symptoms that tend to predict the presence of LOMD. These are gas, bloating, constipation and diarrhea.

Most of us have experienced one or all of these at one time or another. If any that I've listed occur for a very short time (I mean days), or if there is a clear cause for the issue (like perhaps eating unusual food in a foreign country) and the situation resolves quickly, there is no need for concern.

However, in our Western society, in the decades that I've worked with clients, I've found that many people experience one, if not a few, of these uncomfortable symptoms ongoingly. And they think they are "normal." They are sorely mistaken. Signs like these are NOT NORMAL!

> **Listen up - If you have regular gas, bloating, constipation, or diarrhea, that is a sign you most likely are experiencing LOMD and may be headed toward the beginning stages of declining health.**

If I achieve only one goal in this book, it would be to make you aware of the ways your gut attempts to communicate with you to help maintain balance and vitality for all your days.

I don't mean to scare you at all! When I speak of "chronic" symptoms, I mean a minor discomfort that has persisted for a couple of weeks at least. I am not talking about serious issues here, like copious watery diarrhea or intense pain in your chest after eating. These conditions require medical attention.

The conditions in this chapter have two aspects in common:

- They occur in the presence of an imbalance of beneficial to pathogenic microbes, which is a precursor to LOMD.
- They present when there is a disruption in the proper movement of food, toxins, and bacteria through the gut and out of the body. This movement is generally known as "gastric motility" or simply "motility." We will be discussing the tremendous importance of motility as we move forward.

Let's focus on these first signs that are almost "under the radar."

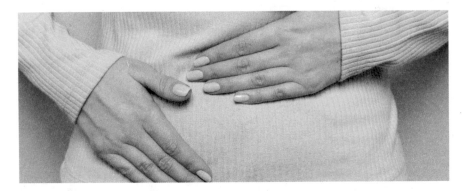

GAS AND BLOATING

Everyone passes gas. And yes, that means you too! The average person passes it approximately 13 times a day.[1] And we have all experienced bloating, that uncomfortable abdominal distention.

Occasional gas and bloating is not generally a reason for alarm or concern, provided that it resolves itself in a day or so. There are several reasons for occasional gas and bloating, including swallowing air, carbonated beverages, eating too quickly, food intolerances to such things as lactose or sucrose, and constipation. At the very least, occasional gas production and abdominal bloating can signal incomplete digestion of food. Many people lack sufficient digestive enzymes, produced by the pancreas, intestinal cells, and, interestingly, gut bacteria, to properly digest the amount and types of food they are eating. Certain foods such as beans, cruciferous vegetables like broccoli and cabbage, and some fruits can be potential problems for some people.

But long-term excess flatulence, belching, and abdominal distention can be one of those "under the radar" signs of bacterial imbalance or LOMD. One critical feature of our intestinal bacteria is that they help us digest our foods. A typical reaction of this digestive process is the production of small amounts of gas such as hydrogen and carbon dioxide. But when the delicate balance of intestinal bacteria becomes disrupted or even worse, specific strains disappear altogether, food starts to ferment while in the intestine, resulting in excess gas production, flatulence, belching, and painful abdominal bloating.

With lower amounts of good bacteria in our guts, harmful bacteria and pathogenic organisms can take hold and upset a healthy gut balance, compounding the problem. When this happens, the reaction of these type of bacteria with food in the small and large intestine produce high amounts of the hydrogen and methane gases, much more so than our good bacteria, resulting in gas and bloating.

What to Do Now

Diet:

Try to limit those foods you may be more sensitive to and which tend to produce more gas, such as beans and cruciferous vegetables. If unsure, try keeping a food diary of what you eat and how you feel several hours later. This practice can help you recognize which foods may be producing more gas.

Supplements:

My first suggestion when it comes to gas and bloating is to take a probiotic supplement and some digestive enzymes with meals to see if this helps resolve the situation. Below is more information regarding what to look for in an enzyme and probiotic formula.

Digestive Enzyme: Look for an enzyme formula that contains higher levels of at least the three essential enzymes outlined below. Take the enzymes just before eating any regular meal or foods you know may cause you gas and bloating.

- At least 100,000 units of protease to help break down proteins
- At least 25,000 units of amylase to help break down carbohydrates
- At least 5,000 units of lipase to help break down fats

In addition to the previous three basic enzymes, several others can be beneficial if included in the formula:

- **Alpha Galactosidase** – helps digest beans and legumes
- **Lactase** – helps digest lactose from dairy - make sure it has this if you are lactose intolerant
- **Cellulase** – helps digest the cellulose of plant cell walls (vegetables and fruits)
- **DDP-IV** – helps to digest gluten – make sure it has this if you know you are gluten intolerant (This does not include being diagnosed with celiac disease. In that case, you must avoid gluten in the diet altogether.)

If you find that you are especially sensitive to lactose or gluten, you can find those specific enzymes by themselves in a stronger dosage.

Probiotics: Helping to re-establish not only the bacterial count but also the bacterial diversity is of utmost importance, so look for a high potency AND high diversity probiotic that contains:

- At least 60 billion probiotic cultures per capsule - this is the potency
- At least 60 unique probiotic strains per capsule - this is the strain diversity
- Both Lactobacillus and Bifidobacterium strains of bacteria
- Prebiotics to supply food for the probiotics

In addition, make sure the supplement uses some form of delayed-release technology so that the probiotics are delivered into the intestine, not the stomach, where they can be destroyed by stomach acid. A delayed-release probiotic capsule can be taken any time of day, with or without food. Also, be sure the potency is guaranteed to date of expiration, not just from the time of manufacture.

Probiotics and digestive enzymes are NOT the same things. Probiotics are the beneficial bacteria that reside in and on the body and in some cases, help to produce enzymes. Digestive enzymes are catalysts that help break our food down into micronutrients.

The addition of both digestive enzymes and a high diversity probiotic can go a long way to help resolve gas and bloating related to LOMD.

DIARRHEA

As I'm sure you are aware of and have experienced at one time or another, diarrhea is the passage of loose, watery stool. It can occur for many reasons, including food poisoning, food sensitivities, laxative abuse, alcohol abuse, even emotional stress.

Diarrhea may be either acute or chronic. Acute diarrhea takes the form of an isolated incident caused by a temporary problem—usually an infection that lasts three to seven days. Chronic diarrhea is much more complex with a multitude of causes and can last for months. A situation involving chronic diarrhea can become severe, especially in the very old and very young.

Once LOMD has started to take hold in your intestinal tract, the lack of strain diversity and an overall abundance of negative gut bacteria may leave you susceptible to intestinal irritation and diarrhea-causing pathogens, such as E. coli, Shigella, and Clostridium difficile. This lack of intestinal protection also can lend itself to parasitic infections like Cryptosporidium or Giardia. Once in the system, pathogenic organisms and parasites produce toxic substances that can further create abnormal gut function, leading to diarrhea.[2] A healthy gut microbiome helps clear such pathogens out of your system before they can cause you such distress.

Conversely, diarrhea onset from something other than LOMD can lead to a microbial imbalance and the start of a vicious cycle.

With any diarrhea situation, the quick passage of intestinal contents results in the inability to absorb many of the needed nutrients that nourish the body. Malabsorption can lead to weakness, brain fog, and nutrient deficiency health issues.

What to Do Now

Diet:

To avoid dehydration, drink plenty of broths, teas, and electrolyte water supplements. Drink rice water by boiling 1 cup brown rice with 5 cups water. Strain and drink liquid throughout the day. Save rice and add to the diet. Bananas are also helpful as they are high in potassium, a mineral lost with dehydration, sometimes as a result of chronic diarrhea.

Supplements:

Fiber: This may be surprising to some, but fiber in supplement form can be very beneficial for those dealing with diarrhea. More notably, soluble fiber which is typically found in foods such as oats and rice bran. Soluble fiber helps absorb the excess liquid and slow things down in the digestive tract. Look for a fiber supplement that includes:

- At least 6 grams of soluble fiber per serving

> **There is a big misconception regarding fiber being a laxative. Fiber itself is not a laxative. The type of fiber taken can help either diarrhea or constipation. Fiber is a regulator of bowel elimination.**

Probiotics: Improving the balance of gut microbiota is imperative with any diarrhea situation, whether acute or chronic. Again, you not only want to re-establish the bacterial count but also the bacterial diversity, so look for a high potency AND high strain diversity probiotic that contains:

- At least 60 billion probiotic cultures per capsule - this is the potency
- At least 60 unique probiotic strains per capsule - this is the strain diversity
- Both Lactobacillus and Bifidobacterium strains of bacteria
- Prebiotics to supply food for the probiotics

In addition, make sure the supplement uses some form of delayed-release technology so that the probiotic delivers into the intestinal system and not the stomach, where it can be destroyed. With delayed-release, you may take the probiotic any time of day, with or without food. Also, make sure the potency is guaranteed to the end of expiration and not only at the time of manufacture.

Saccharomyces boulardii: S. boulardii is a beneficial yeast organism that has been prescribed for diarrheal diseases for over 25 years. It effectively helps modulate the internal ecosystem, helping to restore homeostasis. It has also been shown to interfere with a pathogenic organism's ability to colonize and irritate the intestinal lining. Look for one that contains:

- At least 6 billion cultures per capsule

CONSTIPATION

It seems there are differences in opinion as to what constitutes the definition of constipation. In conventional medical circles, professionals deem it normal to have a bowel movement as infrequently as three times a week.[3] In contrast, most holistic practitioners would consider the normal range of bowel movements to be at least one per day.

Additionally, constipation is recognized by some as incomplete bowel movements, often characterized by stools that are hard, dry, and difficult to pass due to slow transit time through the gastrointestinal tract. The amount of feces eliminated in the bowel movement is another marker of constipation. A daily bowel movement of approximately one and a half feet, which is about the length of the left side of the colon, would be considered normal by natural health practitioners.

There can be numerous contributing factors to constipation, including dehydration, thyroid issues, stress, medication side effects, lack of exercise, lack of fiber in the diet, and nutrient deficiencies such as magnesium and B vitamins. However, one of the most common factors related to ongoing constipation is a disruption in the bacterial ecosystem within the small intestine and colon, which you now know of as LOMD.

As you also know by now, the bacteria in our gut play a crucial role in intestinal health overall and in our gut motility, mentioned earlier in this chapter. Many good bacterial strains produce by-products or metabolites (lactate and short-chain fatty acids) that help control the proper pH of our colonic environment. This pH, meaning the acidity or alkalinity of the colon, is a significant stimulator of good peristaltic movement that results in healthy bowel elimination.

Whereas good bacteria create beneficial metabolites, bad bacteria produce harmful metabolites that result in the exact opposite effect in the colon. They disrupt the pH balance, which can slow down gut motility, resulting in constipation.

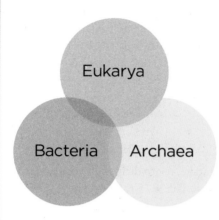

As you learned in Chapter 1, various microbes in the gut can be beneficial, commensal (neutral), or pathogenic (harmful) to the human gut.

All life on earth is classified into three domains:
- Eukarya
- Bacteria
- Archaea

Eukarya can be unicellular (one cell) or multicellular (many cells), and they possess a definite cell nucleus (the control center of a cell). This classification includes fungus, parasites, and protozoa. They can be beneficial, commensal or pathogenic, depending on their type and population. By the way, humans, plants, and animals are all eukaryotes.

Bacteria are unicellular and do not have a nucleus. They beneficially provide productive health benefits in and on the human body. For example, the probiotics Lactobacillus and Bifidobacteria found in the gut belong to this group. There are also commensal and pathogenic bacteria in our intestinal tracts.

Archaea are ancient unicellular microbes, only recently distinguished in form and function from bacteria. Like bacteria, they do not have a nucleus. Archaea can survive in extreme environments and are also typically found at low levels in the human gut and were considered commensal. However, recent research is associating higher levels of archaea with several digestive issues and they now may be considered more pathogenic.[4]

Archaea are "methanogens" and they are the highest producers of methane on the planet. Studies have associated increased methane with chronic constipation, diverticulosis, and other motility issues like IBS that we will explore shortly.

Methane produced by cattle is now documented as a toxic contributor to the greenhouse effect on our world.

Many studies show a distinct difference in bacterial composition in people with chronic constipation compared to those with regular daily elimination. Within the colon microbiome, a decrease in certain types of good bacterial strains is seen, specifically Lactobacillus and Bifidobacterium. There is also an increase in less desirable stains.* Say it with me now - "Lack Of Microbial Diversity" = LOMD!

What to Do Now

Diet:

Try to drink enough water daily. How much is enough? Unless you have a medical condition that restricts water intake, try to drink half your body weight in ounces per day. For example - 150 lbs. X .5 = 75 ounces = how much water to drink per day.

Include foods that are higher in fiber content, such as prunes, pears, and lots of vegetables of any kind. Avoid processed, refined foods such as white bread, white potatoes, cakes, cookies, and fast food.

Supplements:

Natural Laxative Formulation: The idea behind this chapter is to get to the root of why you have constipation, but in the meantime, having a natural laxative formula on hand can be helpful and offer more immediate relief. Look for one that includes:

- Magnesium Hydroxide as the main ingredient
- Other ingredients may consist of cape aloe, rhubarb root, slippery elm bark, and triphala

Fiber: Like with diarrhea, increasing fiber intake can be very advantageous. This time you want to look for a supplement that contains more of the insoluble type of fiber. Insoluble fiber attracts water into your stool, making it easier to pass. It will also speed up the passage of food through the colon, adding bulk to help increase motility. Look for a fiber supplement that contains:

- At least 11 grams of insoluble fiber per serving from ingredients like flaxseed, pea fiber, and hemp fiber. Start slowly with half dosage and build up to full dosage during the first week.

Probiotics: Just as with diarrhea, improving the balance of gut microbiota is imperative. And this bears repeating - you not only want to re-establish the bacterial count but also the bacterial diversity, so look for a high potency AND high strain diversity probiotic that contains:

- At least 60 billion probiotic cultures per capsule - this is the potency
- At least 60 unique probiotic strains per capsule - this is the strain diversity
- Both Lactobacillus and Bifidobacterium strains of bacteria
- Prebiotics to supply food for the probiotics

 Products that contain senna, cascara, or artificial laxatives can be harsh on the intestinal system.

In addition, make sure the supplement uses some form of delayed-release technology so that the probiotic delivers into the intestinal system and not the stomach, where it can be destroyed. With delayed-release, you may take the probiotic any time of day, with or without food. Also, make sure the potency is guaranteed to the end of expiration and not only until the time of manufacture.

Look for a probiotic that offers a large amount of Bifidobacteria cultures and strains per serving. Bifidobacterium is the most noted and needed type of bacteria in the colon, where constipation occurs.

Hopefully, the suggestions made for those experiencing the onset of gas and bloating, diarrhea, or constipation, or all of these, will help turn your gut around and get you back into proper balance quickly. If not, keep reading on to Chapter 6, as you may have more than just the First Signs.

TO RECAP:

- Gas, bloating, diarrhea, or constipation should not be considered normal digestive processes.

- If you have regular gas, bloating, diarrhea, or constipation you may be advancing toward declining health.

- Helpful suggestions include digestive enzymes, probiotics, fiber, and occasional use of a natural laxative.

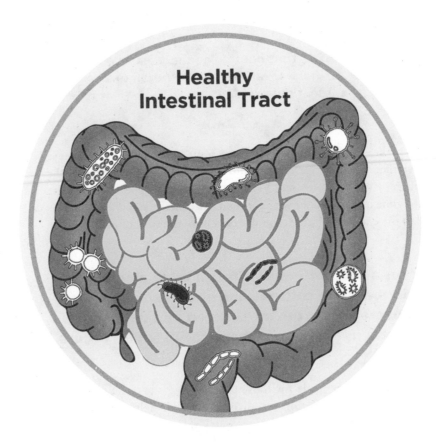

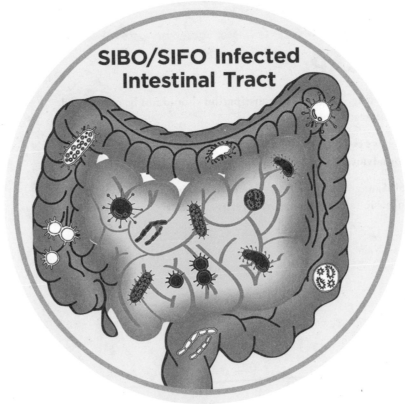

CHAPTER 6

IBS-COULD IT BE MORE?
SIBO/SIFO/GERD

Let's have a quick review. In Chapter 5, I described the first signs of LOMD. They are gas and bloating, diarrhea or constipation, or all of these together! Most importantly, I wanted you to clearly understand that although these issues are prevalent in Western society, they are NOT NORMAL when experienced day after day!

If you are one of those people who have "tried everything," even many of the suggestions that I offered in the last chapter, then this following information may be precisely what you've been waiting to hear! There can be relief! Vibrant health can be restored!

IT'S TIME TO DISCUSS CONDITIONS KNOWN AS
SIBO AND SIFO - Small Intestinal Bacterial Overgrowth and Small Intestinal Fungal Overgrowth

In previous chapters, we focused on the development of LOMD in relation to the colon (large intestine) environment where, you now know, most of our beneficial bacteria reside. However, when LOMD continues to develop over time, creating an unhealthy colon environment, it can soon start to affect the upper GI tract as well, impacting the small intestine and even as far up as the stomach.

Bacteria species can start to ascend upward into the small intestine, which typically houses very few bacteria and presents a different microbial makeup than the colon. Once in the small intestine, they thrive on available food that they did not have in the colon, setting off a full-blown disruption to the microbial complex within the small intestine. This overgrowth is known as SIBO or Small Intestinal Bacterial Overgrowth.

> **For years previous, doctors labeled people with symptoms of SIBO as having IBS – Irritable Bowel Syndrome. Although other situations such as food poisoning can cause IBS, it is now estimated that 40-70 percent of people diagnosed with IBS actually have SIBO.**

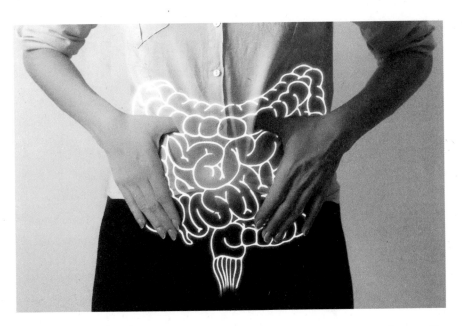

Once there, the displaced bacteria and the environment it creates can often enable the growth of fungal organisms. Abnormal fungal growth is now known as SIFO or Small Intestinal Fungal Overgrowth and often accompanies the diagnosis of SIBO. The most noted fungal organism that tends to take root in this situation is the organism called Candida. Years ago, we called this situation "Candida Overgrowth," not realizing its relationship to SIBO.

The upward movement of the colonic bacteria (both good and bad) can be exacerbated by several contributing factors. First, there can be a dysfunction of the ileocecal valve, the essential sphincter muscle at the junction of the small and large intestine.[1] ....This "valve" is responsible for letting food matter down into the large intestine and preventing the contents of the large intestine from moving upward into the small intestine. This dysfunction can occur due to gaseous pressure as a result of LOMD within the colonic environment.

Secondly is impaired motility within the gut. I introduced "motility" in Chapter 5 and promised to explain more. Now is the time. Motility describes the mechanism whereby food, toxins, and bacteria are moved downward through the gut and out of the body in elimination. I want to explain two types of motility to you, so please bear with me here.

The first is called peristalsis. Most people know this type of motility as happening shortly after eating to help propel food down the intestinal tract. Peristalsis occurs within any smooth muscle of the intestinal system, including the esophagus, the stomach, and the small and large intestine.

There is, however, another type of motility called Migrating Motor Complex or MMC for short. MMC is also a contraction but of only the small intestinal tract and happens around 3 hours after meals. Its primary functions are to propel any remaining food in the small intestine downward and sweep the small intestine of bacteria. Remember, the small intestine is not supposed to contain many bacteria. The MMC is one of the ways our body keeps 98% of our bacteria in the colon and helps prevent SIBO in the process.

When our gut motility dysfunctions, especially the MMC type of motility, this can set the stage for the bacteria within the colon to gain easier access upward into the small intestine. The hormone motilin partially stimulates the MMC and is only produced when the stomach is empty. The MMC can malfunction when you do not allow enough time between meals or by laying down too soon after eating before the stomach has had time to empty.

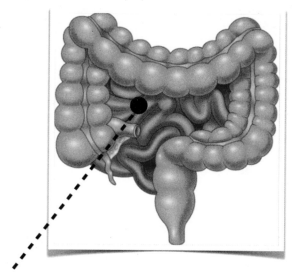

MIGRATING MOTOR COMPLEX
Waves of muscular activity move waste and unwanted bacteria through the digestive tract and on to the colon.

The digestive system is also endowed with its very own nervous system called the Enteric Nervous System (ENS), which helps control the contraction and relaxation of the Migrating Motor Complex. If disorder occurs within this specialized nervous system, digestive havoc can ensue.

Speaking of nerves, one more factor worth mentioning can exacerbate the development of SIBO and SIFO. It involves the vagus nerve. We looked briefly at the vagus nerve in Chapter 3. To recap, the vagus nerve is cranial nerve 10 and is also known as the wandering nerve, as it travels throughout your body, interacting with the organs and tissues.

Although the vagus nerve is involved in many functions within the human body, it is the main pathway for our gut/brain connection. It is the vagus nerve that gives the enteric nervous system its direction. A disruption in the proper function of the vagus nerve can cause a signaling problem for the MMC, resulting in either fast or slow motility, neither ideal. The most common causes of vagus nerve impairment are alcoholism, diabetes, physical or surgical trauma, and tumors.

As you can now see, the gut is a highly complicated organ, and many factors can all work together in creating the perfect storm for SIBO and SIFO to occur. Once the bacterial strains get displaced into the small intestine and/or fungal overgrowth takes place, it can be a long and tedious situation to eradicate.

Symptoms:

The symptoms associated with SIBO and SIFO can be many. Most notably, if extreme abdominal bloating and gas are unresolved with enzymes or by other suggestions offered in our previous chapter, you may have SIBO or SIFO. Other symptoms can include but are not limited to fibromyalgia type aches and pains, brain fog, skin rashes, sleep disturbances, anxiety, depression, food intolerances, constipation, and/or diarrhea.

I would like to expand on the symptom of gas for a bit (no pun intended) and why you may experience either constipation or diarrhea or both intermittently. In the last chapter, you may recall, I described the three domains of organisms found on earth, two of which can be found in the human intestinal system: Bacteria and Archaea. Both of these microorganisms can flourish in a dysbiotic colon and find their way up into the small intestine with SIBO. However, the condition is named Bacterial Overgrowth and not Bacteria/Archaea Overgrowth.

Once abnormally thriving in the small intestine, certain types of bacteria will produce a gas called hydrogen. This gas production, of course, is part of the abdominal gas and distention produced from SIBO. When hydrogen production is high in the intestinal system, a person tends to experience diarrhea.

In the opposite direction, when more Archaea are dominant in the overgrowth, methane gas is produced. When there is a lot of methane produced in the intestinal system, a person tends to experience constipation. Even without SIBO, people who tend to house more of these archaea organisms in their colon can suffer from chronic constipation.

Interestingly, one of the only reliable ways to diagnose SIBO is by measuring the hydrogen and methane gases found in the breath. See Chapter 8 for more information regarding this type of testing.

The longer SIBO and SIFO take place without resolution, the more damage can occur. The infiltration of unwanted organisms can degrade the protective mucus lining of the small intestine, leaving way for the by-products of bacterial overgrowth to enter the bloodstream. One of the primary and most damaging by-products is lipopolysaccharide (LPS). LPS can have a devastating effect on the liver and other organs and tissues throughout the body. Once in the blood, the reaction is a heightened immune and inflammatory response that can cause damage to the blood vessels, the kidneys, the adrenals, and more. At the very least initiating the increased permeability of the intestinal lining, better known as Leaky Gut.

What To Do Now

Diet/Lifestyle:

Suggested diets for SIBO/SIFO can vary depending on who is making the suggestions. Some SIBO specialists will suggest following a low FODMAP diet (fermentable oligosaccharides, disaccharides, monosaccharides, and polyols). These are short-chain carbohydrates and sugar alcohols that are poorly absorbed by the body that may cause excessive gas, bloating, and abdominal pain. This diet can be very restrictive, and some doctors recommend it only for two to three months due to possible resulting nutritional deficiencies.

What is essential to know is that while trying to eradicate SIBO/SIFO, you must avoid foods that can contribute to the fermentation of the misplaced bacteria. This will include but is not limited to:

- Sugar and high sugar foods. Sugar alcohols which are used as sweeteners such as xylitol, sorbitol, maltitol, and erythritol

- Beans, legumes, lentils

- Broccoli, brussels, cauliflower, coleslaw

- Most green plants such as lettuces, kale, collards, etc., except spinach and arugula

- Fermented foods such as kefir, kombucha and sauerkraut

- Higher sugar fruits such as apples, bananas, and grapes

- Dairy-based foods such as yogurt and ice cream

- Wheat-based foods such as cookies, crackers, and breads

- Alcohol

NOTE If any food causes more bloating and discomfort, exclude it during the eradication phase.

Try to stick to foods low on the fermentation scale. This includes mostly all meats (except processed deli meats), fish, eggs, root/fruit type vegetables such as zucchini, squash, beets, carrots, eggplant, green beans, tomato, and peppers. See chapter 9 for more resources regarding a SIBO diet.

Try not to lie down or sleep within 3 hours after eating.

Supplements:

Besides following the SIBO diet and previous suggestions, supplements can be very helpful with SIBO and SIFO.

Bacterial Overgrowth Detox - The first step to help rebalance your gut environment is to find products that can help eliminate bacterial and fungal overgrowth without compounding the issue. Look for a product that contains ingredients such as oregano oil, thyme oil, clove leaf oil, black cumin oil, and cinnamon leaf oil. You may need to take this type of product for several months straight when first starting a program and then periodically after that.

Intestinal Lining Support Product - You also need to make sure to support the integrity of the gut lining with ingredients such as L-glutamine, N-acetyl-glucosamine (non-shellfish sourced), aloe vera, DGL type of licorice extract, ginger, and marshmallow root. Look for a powder formulation that includes these ingredients. Take one scoop daily on empty stomach.

Fiber Supplement - A fiber supplement that is mostly insoluble versus soluble fiber can be helpful to support bowel regularity - both diarrhea and constipation. Look for one that contains flax, pea, and hemp fibers, as these are high in insoluble fiber. Soluble fiber promoted as a prebiotic can contribute to bacterial growth, which is not suggested during a SIBO eradication program.

Probiotic - Although you would think a probiotic supplement would be a leading suggestion, it is not recommended during the initial phase of eradicating bacterial overgrowth. A high potency, high diversity probiotic can be added once the symptoms of SIBO/SIFO have dissipated to help repopulate your good bacteria. When choosing a probiotic supplement, look for a high potency AND high strain diversity probiotic that contains:

- At least 60 billion probiotic cultures per capsule - this is the potency
- At least 60 unique probiotic strains per capsule - this is the strain diversity
- Both Lactobacillus and Bifidobacterium strains of bacteria
- Prebiotics to supply food for the probiotics

GERD

Gastroesophageal reflux disease (GERD) is a condition known by various names, often called acid reflux, chronic heartburn, or acid indigestion. These terms are frequently used in advertisements to get you to buy the latest pill or tablet guaranteed to ease your pain. But if you are experiencing discomfort regularly, recurring heartburn is likely the symptom of a more significant problem.

GERD is a digestive disorder in which partially digested food from the stomach, along with stomach acid, also known as hydrochloric acid (HCl), and enzymes, backs up into the esophagus. This process is known as reflux.

Your stomach acid has a low pH, meaning that it is very acidic. Even if present in low amounts, HCl can cause damage when it comes into contact with the delicate lining of the esophagus.

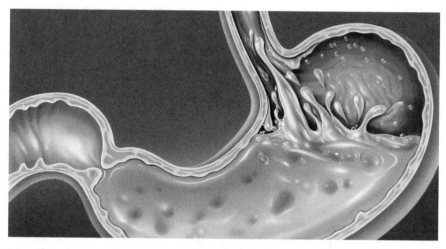

Usually, the lower esophageal sphincter (LES), the muscle that connects the esophagus to the upper portion of the stomach, opens to allow food from the esophagus into the stomach; then, it closes immediately to prevent food and digestive stomach secretions from reentering the esophagus.

Reflux occurs when the LES weakens and malfunctions, staying open after food has entered the stomach and allowing the stomach's contents to flow backward into the esophagus.

There are several reasons this backward flow can occur:
- Overeating
- Eating too quickly
- Eating while stressed
- Lying down after eating
- Tight-fitting clothes
- Hiatal hernia
- Pressure from pregnancy
- Carbonated drinks
- Spicy foods
- Fried and fatty foods

Very commonly, however, it is a motility issue due to pressure from further down the intestinal tract and can easily manifest as a symptom of LOMD and/or SIBO/SIFO.

The pressure that develops within the intestinal system with bacterial imbalance (remember gas and bloating) can create the upward flow of intestinal and stomach contents all the way up to the esophageal area. The mucous lining, or mucosa, of the esophagus, is not designed to withstand the caustic effects of acid, bile, and stomach contents and results in irritation of this delicate lining. Unfortunately, the longer reflux is present and the more irritation that occurs (known as esophagitis), the more likely a resulting condition called Barrett's esophagus can develop, considered a precancerous situation.

With SIBO or SIFO, as we described, LOMD and bacterial imbalance along with motility issues (remember I mention lying down after eating above?) can also create pressure and result in GERD. Poor dietary choices only fuel the discomfort.

Choosing medications to alleviate the burning sensations temporarily adds to imbalances in the entire digestive system, as you learned in Chapter 2, and magnifies GERD over time. Sadly, GERD is one of the most common digestive issues experienced in our society and points to developing LOMD.

> **We Need Stomach Acid! While acid-suppressing drugs may offer temporary relief, long-term usage has been shown to contribute to the development of pneumonia, dementia, osteoporosis, B-12 deficiency, and interestingly enough, hypergastrinemia (rebound overproduction of stomach acid).**

What To Do Now
Diet/Lifestyle:

Avoid overeating by eating smaller meals more frequently, spaced by at least 3 hours. Avoid fried, fatty, and spicy foods. Do not eat any later than 3 hours before bed or lie down immediately after eating. Loosen the beltline on clothing or wear loose-fitting clothing.

Supplements:

It is crucial to make sure that you are protecting the delicate esophageal lining and digesting your food sufficiently with GERD. You can also follow the suggestions made in the SIBO/SIFO section, as GERD can result from that situation.

Esophageal Lining Support Product - Make sure to support the integrity of the esophageal lining with ingredients such as L-glutamine, N-acetyl-glucosamine (non-shellfish sourced), aloe vera, DGL type of licorice extract, ginger, and marshmallow root. Look for a powder formulation that includes these ingredients. Take one scoop daily on an empty stomach.

Digestive Enzyme: Look for an enzyme formula that contains higher levels of at least the three basic enzymes as outlined below. In addition, you can find an enzyme formula that includes hydrochloric acid (stomach acid) in the form of Betaine HCl. Take the enzymes with any regular meal or foods you know may cause you discomfort. Do not take an HCl supplement on an empty stomach or if you have a current stomach ulcer.

- At least 100,000 units of protease to help break down proteins
- At least 25,000 units of amylase to help break down carbohydrates
- At least 5,000 units of lipase to help break down fats
- Betaine HCL - 500 to 600 mg per capsule to support stomach acid

Probiotics: Improving the balance of gut microbiota is imperative with GERD. Again, you want to re-establish the bacterial count and the bacterial diversity, so look for a high potency AND high strain diversity probiotic that contains:

- At least 60 billion probiotic cultures per capsule - this is the potency
- At least 60 unique probiotic strains per capsule - this is the strain diversity
- Both Lactobacillus and Bifidobacterium strains of bacteria
- Prebiotics to supply food for the probiotics

In addition, make sure the supplement uses some form of delayed-release technology so that the probiotic delivers into the intestinal system and not the stomach, where it can be destroyed. With a delayed-release capsule, you may take the probiotic any time of day, with or without food. Also, make sure the potency is guaranteed to end of expiration and not at the time of manufacture.

NOTE

If taking probiotics to manage GERD increases intestinal discomfort, please discontinue and follow the SIBO/SIFO suggestions.

Concerning the resolution of GERD, I realize you want one answer on how to resolve this issue. Each of us is unique, and, as with other digestive problems, it often is a matter of trial and error. Don't give up!

TO RECAP:

- If having continued digestive discomfort or diagnosed with IBS, consider you may have SIBO/SIFO.

- Bacteria migration into the small intestine can be due to:
  - Ileocecal valve dysfunction
  - Migrating Motor Complex dysfunction
  - Vagus nerve disruption

- Chronic GERD or reflux can be a resulting factor of SIBO or LOMD

- Helpful suggestions include to follow a low FODMAP diet, and supplements such as bacterial overgrowth detox, intestinal lining support product, insoluble fiber, digestive enzymes and probiotics.

LOMD and Declining Health

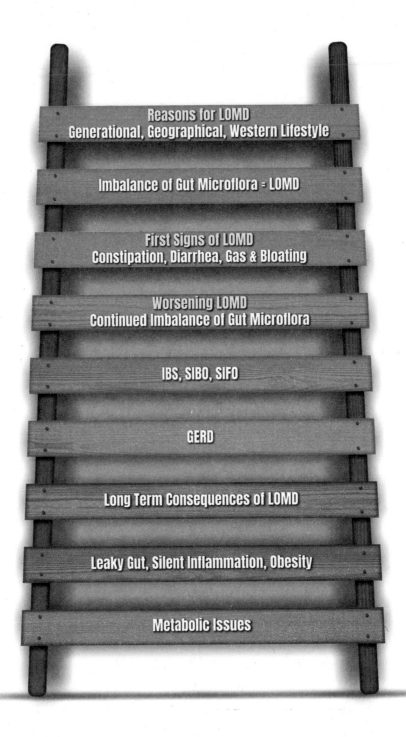

Reasons for LOMD
Generational, Geographical, Western Lifestyle

Imbalance of Gut Microflora = LOMD

First Signs of LOMD
Constipation, Diarrhea, Gas & Bloating

Worsening LOMD
Continued Imbalance of Gut Microflora

IBS, SIBO, SIFO

GERD

Long Term Consequences of LOMD

Leaky Gut, Silent Inflammation, Obesity

Metabolic Issues

CHAPTER 7

LOMD AND LONG-TERM CONSEQUENCES OF INFLAMMATION

By now, I'm sure you're beginning to get the idea that LOMD is a very serious health concern. One of the most challenging aspects of health is that it is actually "silent" in many cases. We've discussed obvious symptoms like gas and bloating, constipation, diarrhea, and actual pains in the gut resulting from microbial imbalance associated with LOMD, many times referred to as "dysbiosis." We've also discussed SIBO/SIFO and GERD along with their telltale symptoms.

What about situations that don't give us any "warning signs"?

I'd like to address that rung of declining health in this chapter. I'm not sharing this information to scare you or to have you imagining issues at each turn. Instead, I'd like to offer you an understanding of the process of declining health, ultimately along with a pretty simple "to-do" list that will support your best life as you age.

I wrote a 430-page book a few years ago called *Heart of Perfect Health*. At the core of my message at that time was how a condition called "silent inflammation" leads to the types of issues we may experience as we age. Commonly faced is the potential for metabolic problems like high blood pressure, high cholesterol, cardiovascular conditions, and blood sugar issues, often not discovered until they are well established.

Sadly, in our society, these types of issues are emerging in much younger people than in the past. Often, they are associated with obesity, which we will address shortly. All of these conditions too often have their beginnings in the gut. So let's explore together.

We've all heard of "inflammation." Healthy inflammation is part of the body's natural repair process. It's our first-line defense against injury and infection. However, when inflammation originates in the gut, it may enter into total body circulation and initiate problems far from where it started.

Leaky Gut

Damage from gut toxins to the delicate intestinal lining can set the stage for increased permeability or "leaky gut," a central component of silent inflammation. We've made mention of leaky gut already in several places in this book. Let's take a closer look.

DIGESTIVE CARE

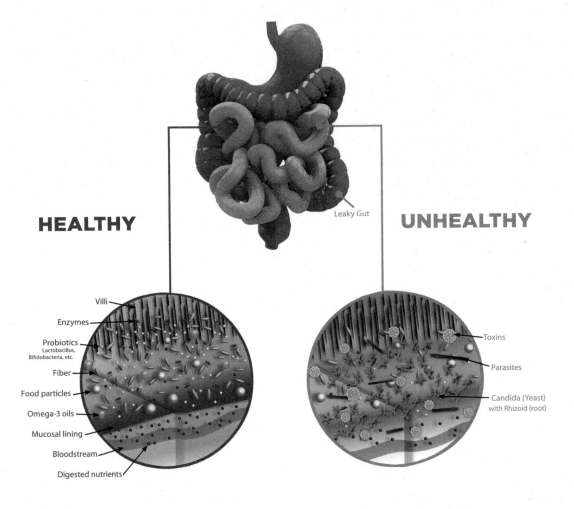

HEALTHY

Leaky Gut

UNHEALTHY

Villi
Enzymes
Probiotics
Lactobacillus,
Bifidobacteria, etc.
Fiber
Food particles
Omega-3 oils
Mucosal lining
Bloodstream
Digested nutrients

Toxins
Parasites
Candida (Yeast)
with Rhizoid (root)

LEAKY GUT

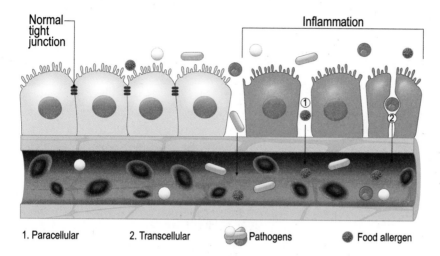

1. Paracellular   2. Transcellular   Pathogens   Food allergen

The intestinal lining is a one-cell-thick layer that separates the intestine and contents from the entire blood circulation. That's right, one-cell-thick! This layer is like your skin, delineating the inside of your body from the outside. Technically, proteins, carbs, fats, vitamins, and other substances are only considered to have entered the body once they pass through the intestinal lining. Only the tiniest food particles, nutrients, and substances should be able to pass through the gut lining into circulation.

Think of your intestinal lining as a screen, letting in fresh air but keeping out mosquitoes. When the screen has a hole, unwanted insects can get in. Leaky gut is like having a screen with holes - allowing unwanted particles to pass through the lining into your body! Leaky gut opens a gateway into the body for toxins, undigested food particles, and bacteria to enter circulation. Silent inflammation is a response by the immune system to this constant influx of foreign invaders.

> **As we learned in Chapter 3, probiotics can help maintain intestinal barrier function as one of their 8 primary purposes.**

"Endotoxemia" is a technical name for the presence of harmful bacterial toxins (endotoxins) in the bloodstream. Endotoxins are harmful substances produced inside the body, as compared to exotoxins which come from our environment. Endotoxins tend to initiate generalized "low-grade inflammation."[1] Frequently it is endotoxins produced by the various microbes that stimulate inflammation rather than the microbes themselves.

In the previous chapter, we mentioned one extremely damaging endotoxin called LPS. LPS is a cell wall component of certain intestinal bacteria, shed when the bacteria die in the intestines. (Bacteria have a short lifespan and are constantly reproducing in the intestines). One way that LPS enters the bloodstream is through a leaky gut.

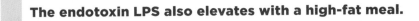

The endotoxin LPS also elevates with a high-fat meal.

As LOMD exacerbates and microbial imbalance magnifies, the possibility of leaky gut mounts, and with it, the probability of toxins "leaking" into the rest of the body.

Also, keep in mind that up to 80 percent of the immune system resides in the gut, so immune responses throughout the body may be impacted by gut inflammation, triggering issues like allergies and food sensitivities.

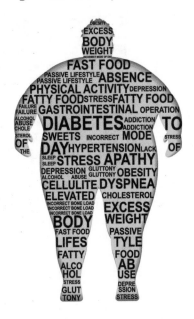

Obesity

Obesity is a condition that haunts, overwhelms, and frustrates our society. It is so pervasive that our society now seems to celebrate the condition. I love all of our people, and I have no issue with anyone who is obese. However, what disturbs me is the number of overweight people that I've met with serious health issues. The U.S. adult obesity rate stands at 42.4 percent, the first time the national rate has passed the 40 percent mark. The national adult obesity rate has increased by 26 percent since 2008.[2]

Particularly distressing to me is the effect obesity is having on our youth. The latest National Health and Nutrition Examination Survey, published in January 2021, reports that about 19 percent of children and adolescents in the U.S. are obese. They call this a record high.[3] This statistic makes me want to cry.

Please understand, silent inflammation, leaky gut, and obesity go hand in hand, setting the stage for high blood pressure, type 2 diabetes, cardiovascular and immune issues. More commonly than ever, these issues once considered "conditions for the aged," are occurring in our youth with startling frequency.

There are several different ways that obesity is determined, however for our discussion, let's agree that obesity is the accumulation of body fat. So, what drives this fat accumulation?

Most people think it's the result of an imbalance between the amount of energy consumed (as food) and the amount of energy expended (as physical activity). However, the truth is much more complicated than that.

METABOLIC INFLUENCES THAT RESULT IN OBESITY
- **Diet**
- **Hormonal influences**
- **Certain medical conditions**
- **Various medications**
- **Age**
- **Environmental toxins**
- **GUT FUNCTION!**

In the other books I've written and earlier in this one, I've explored metabolic influences from different perspectives. Today, I'll discuss how obesity is far too often the result of LOMD and impaired gut function.

In my book, Skinny Gut Diet, I reported on some of the first scientific studies to uncover the gut connection to obesity.

At the core, the research revealed that overall bacterial diversity was decreased (LOMD) in those who were overweight versus those who were lean.

More specifically, certain groups of the bacterial species were increased, and others were reduced in both obese mice and humans compared to lean individuals.[4,5,6]

In other words, the difference in bacterial balance was not only the result of being fat or of eating an obesity-inducing diet but also plays a causative role in weight gain. That is, having the wrong balance of bacteria in your gut can make you fat. And having the right balance of gut bacteria can protect you from getting fat. Have I piqued your interest?

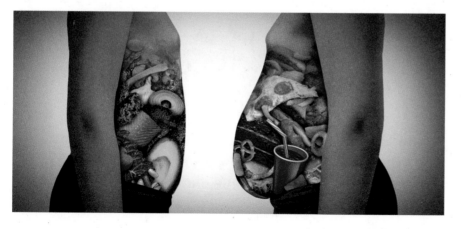

I was so excited that these discoveries led me to create our own in-house research study and write *The Skinny Gut Diet* book. With our cohort of 10 participants, we tracked beneficial, commensal, and pathogenic bacteria levels, and in particular, we observed communities of the two groups mentioned earlier. Their genus names are Firmicutes and Bacteriodetes, which we nicknamed "Fat bacteria" and "Be skinny bacteria," respectively.

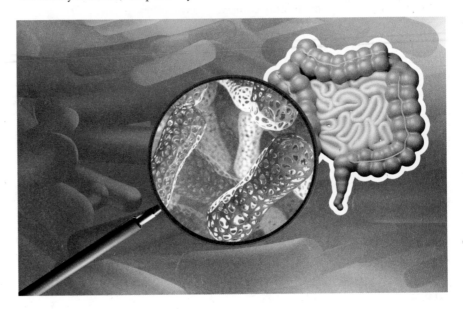

Interestingly, Fat bacteria can harvest more energy from food than the Be skinny bacteria.[7] This was initially discovered when lean mice were colonized with gut bacteria from obese mice and rapidly gained weight within the next 10 to 14 days despite decreased food consumption.[8] Conversely, colonizing obese mice with the bacteria from lean mice initialized weight loss. It appears that the more Fat bacteria you have, the more weight you tend to accumulate.

At this point, you may be wondering - what comes first, the obesity or the gut imbalance? One exciting study addressed this question directly and found that a change in gut balance clearly preceded weight gain.[9]

Researchers from Finland investigating the link between gut bacteria and health wanted to know if an infant's gut bacterial composition could predict the later development of obesity. This multi-year study compared stool samples from overweight or obese children to those of normal-weight children. They discovered significantly higher numbers of beneficial Bifidobacteria in the infants who ended up normal-weight at seven years compared to those children who ended up overweight.[10]

Bifidobacteria are well known for providing health benefits, including reduced gut inflammation (leaky gut), gut lining support, and improved immune function.

They also found higher amounts of S. aureus in the overweight children. S. aureus is a pathogenic bacteria that triggers low-grade inflammation, leading to obesity. Remember my earlier reference to the relationship of gut imbalance, leaky gut, and silent inflammation to obesity?

Please bear with me for one more impactful study. These same Finnish researchers found that gut microbe composition differs between overweight and normal-weight pregnant women.[11] In addition, the gut bacteria not only contribute to weight gain in pregnant mothers but also predict the later development of obesity in children born to these mothers!

Here's the deal. Gut imbalance contributes to weight gain during pregnancy. The mothers then pass the bacteria on to their infants, who later become overweight. Subsequently, those overweight children are more likely to become overweight adults.

Hold on, don't feel overwhelmed. Fortunately, there is a backup system for improving the balance of gut bacteria for your infant - nature's perfect food, breast milk. Breast milk contains the ideal nutrients for babies that promote the growth of beneficial bacteria, as long as the mother is well nourished.

If you're considering pregnancy and find this information interesting, please pick up a copy of *The Skinny Gut Diet*, and give your beautiful babe their best chance for a healthy gut and life!

Additionally, before you begin to fret that your gut bacteria are destined for imbalance because of factors surrounding your birth and upbringing, rest assured that you can restore balance to your gut with the help of probiotic supplements and an appropriate diet. *The Skinny Gut Diet*, along with this book and our resources, can show you how.

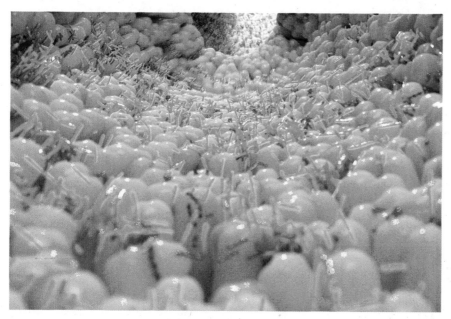

At this point, let's take a quick look at some more wide-ranging effects of obesity that may be impacting you or those you love today. Did you know that today "fat tissue," aka "adipose tissue," is considered an endocrine organ that plays a significant role in metabolism? [12]

Fat tissue secretes a variety of molecules, known as adepokines, which send signals to distant systems of the body. Fat cells also contain receptors that receive signals from different systems of the body. Together these functions classify fat tissue as an organ! We all have fat tissue, and actually, body fat in all of us plays a major role in regulating insulin sensitivity (blood sugar balance).

However, not all fat is the same. The most concerning fat is belly fat, the fat surrounding the organs inside the abdomen. Belly fat is also known as "visceral adipose tissue" (VAT), and that is the one fat you don't want to have. VAT is the most metabolically active fat in the body and contributes to chronic silent inflammation, underlying heart disease, and many other metabolic issues.

Metabolic Issues

As I've mentioned previously, high blood pressure, cardiovascular conditions like atherosclerosis, blood sugar issues, and arthritis (yes, arthritis too) can be unpleasant results of silent inflammation. Indeed, obesity is included as a metabolic issue as well, although we've discussed it separately.

One widespread example is atherosclerosis. Silent inflammation damages the walls of the blood vessels, attracting white blood cells along with fat and calcium. This intricate process leads to "hardening of the arteries," which is the precursor to many other cardiovascular issues. Fortunately, this process is reversible. [13]

 Gut inflammation is recognized as a contributor to the development of heart disease.[14]

VICIOUS CIRCLE

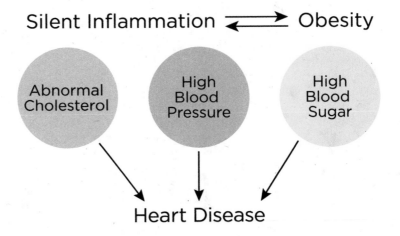

The Bottom Line

Toxins flowing through your circulation (where they are not supposed to be!) can wreak havoc throughout the body, many times without discernible symptoms resulting in silent inflammation. And these toxins gain access through a leaky gut. What a vicious circle!

LOMD and declining health over time is not a one-way ladder. Depending on many factors (age, diet, genetics, and environmental situations), the repercussions of LOMD can manifest at almost any age and any point, although undoubtedly cumulative issues as you age are the most common.

Do not be discouraged. Fortunately, reversing LOMD and supporting your gut health along with your overall well-being is not a difficult process. Admittedly, you will have to make some adjustments to your current lifestyle. However, restoring gut balance can be a fulfilling and rewarding journey, resulting in vibrant health and vitality.

Chronic low-grade inflammation has been associated with high blood pressure and is now known to precede its development.[15]

TO RECAP:

- One of the major long-term consequences of Loss of Microbial Diversity (LOMD) is a condition called "silent inflammation."

- Silent inflammation can lead to metabolic problems such as high blood pressure, high cholesterol, and cardiovascular issues.

- The development of intestinal permeability, better known as leaky gut, from long-term LOMD can be the epicenter of silent inflammation.

- Silent inflammation, leaky gut, and obesity go hand in hand, setting the stage for more long-term health issues.

- Fortunately, reversing LOMD and supporting your gut health along with your overall well-being is not a difficult process.

THE HEALTH CONTINUUM

OPTIMUM HEALTH

- High Energy
- Ideal Weight
- Re-establish Gut Microbiome - Probiotics
- Repair Intestinal Lining
- Detox & Cleanse Intestinal System
- Improved Diet
- Awareness and Education

WHICH WAY ARE YOU HEADING?

- Lack of Awareness
- Imbalance of Gut Microflora - LOMD
- First Signs - Gas & Bloating, Constipation, Diarrhea
- Continued Imbalance of Microbiome
- SIBO/SIFO, GERD
- Long-term Consequences and Silent Inflammation
- Leaky Gut, Obesity, Metabolic Issues

CHRONIC ILL HEALTH

CHAPTER 8

SIMPLE SOLUTIONS

This chapter aims to provide you with general guidelines concerning diet, lab testing, supplementation, and alternative therapies. I believe this could prove helpful in your quest for a healthier microbiome. However, I feel that working through a more serious situation such as LOMD and especially SIBO/SIFO, leaky gut, and the associated health issues warrants having an integrative practitioner familiar with gut health. They can offer appropriate types of testing such as those listed below and guide you through treatment.

Need assistance finding an integrative practitioner? We have found these sources to be very helpful over the years:

The Institute for Functional Medicine: www.ifm.org
American Association of Naturopathic Physicians: https://naturopathic.org
Academy of Integrative Health & Medicine: https://aihm.org
Bastyr University: https://bastyr.edu/Practitioner
FON Consulting Advanced Integrative Medicine has a resource list of clinics: https://fonconsulting.com/resources/integrative-medicine-centers/

I also suggest speaking with your local health food stores as they can be acquainted with natural health practitioners in your immediate area.

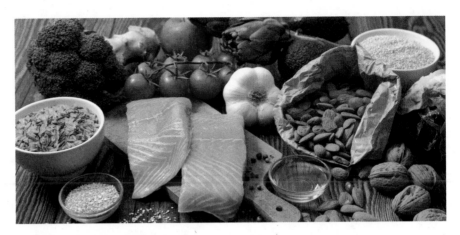

DIET AND LIFESTYLE

For General Gut Health:

Practically speaking, a common-sense quality eating plan can best promote intestinal and overall well-being. Choose organic when possible. I suggest a predominately grain-free diet, avoiding processed, refined, or GMO products completely. Processed, refined grains have been shown to contribute to an upregulated inflammatory response in the body. Refined grains such as white flour, white bread, and white rice have fiber and many nutrients removed during the milling process. If you are intent on eating grains, be sure you choose organic whole grains such as brown rice, wild rice, barley, quinoa, steel-cut oats, as well as sprouted grains and seeds.

Including a large portion of plant-based foods daily is beneficial for cardiovascular, gut, and overall health. Plants contain antioxidants, vitamins, minerals, and fiber that can act as the food source for your good intestinal bacteria (remember prebiotics?). Eat generous amounts of dark green leafy vegetables, peppers, bean sprouts, green peas, spinach, carrots, sweet corn, asparagus, artichokes, brussels sprouts, mushrooms, and broccoli, as well as soaked beans and legumes.

For those who love fruits, it's best to limit high-sugar fruits such as bananas, raisins, grapes, and mangoes to avoid blood sugar spikes. Regularly choose lower-sugar fruit with high fiber content such as blackberries, blueberries, raspberries, and green apples.

Healthy fats are necessary to any diet and include Omega-3 fatty acids derived from salmon, walnuts, avocado, chia, and flax seeds. High-quality extra virgin olive oil is also a valuable and delicious addition to any eating plan.

In my book, *The Skinny Gut Diet*, I lay out a delicious and convenient eating plan accompanied by simple and tasty recipes. Although this book is geared toward weight loss, it also details how to eat for better bacterial balance in the gut. Another book I've mentioned, *Heart of Perfect Health*, has delicious heart and gut-healthy recipes with full graphic instructions. You can find both of these books available for purchase at www.brendawatson.com or at online retailers.

SIBO Diet:

If you suspect or have been told you have SIBO or SIFO (remember, they may be called Candida or IBS), follow the more specific diet recommendations listed in Chapter 6 under SIBO/SIFO. You can find additional information on various acceptable foods and diets to follow on websites such as:

www.sibocenter.com

www.siboinfo.com

www.sibosurvivor.com

www.vitalfoodtherapeutics.com

NOTE

Whenever you follow an elimination diet for any reason, be gentle in re-introducing foods back into your diet. Proceed slowly, adding back one food at a time per week. Take note of how you react to this food before re-introducing another. If the food exacerbates your symptoms, put it back on the shelf, no matter how much you may be craving it! Try again at a later date. Your gut will thank you.

LAB TESTING

Several lab tests may be beneficial in determining the extent of bacterial and digestive issues you may be experiencing. An integrative practitioner typically performs these tests, but some can be found for direct purchase on websites such as: https://www.walkinlab.com

- **Basic Microbiology Stool Analysis** – This type of test will evaluate the levels of beneficial bacteria as well as imbalanced gut bacteria, yeast, and pathogenic organisms. Several labs offer these tests to practitioners, including Genova Diagnostics (Microbiology Analysis) and Doctor's Data (Microbiology Profile or GI 360 Microbiome). The GI 360 Microbiome test also offers a good look at the diversity of your bacterial composition.

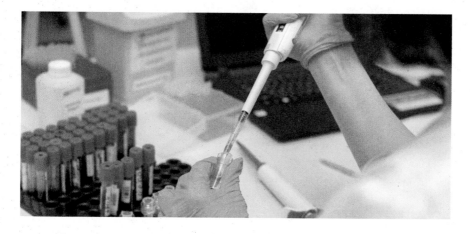

- **Comprehensive Stool Analysis** – A comprehensive stool analysis will offer the same information as the Basic Microbiology Stool Analysis, but in addition will show you more digestive parameters such as inflammatory markers, food digestive markers, parasites, viruses, and gut immunology. There are many stool tests on the market which offer some, or all, of these parameters. We've found the most notable labs offering these tests are Genova Diagnostics (GI Effects Comprehensive Stool Profile) and Doctor's Data (Comprehensive Stool Analysis with Parasitology X 3 or GI 360 Profile). Again, the GI 360 Profile offers a detailed look at the diversity of the bacteria.

- **Intestinal Permeability (Leaky Gut) Test** – This test assesses the small intestine barrier function and absorption of nutrients. It measures the ability of two nonmetabolized sugar molecules to pass through the intestinal mucosa. To perform this test, you must drink a mix of lactulose and mannitol and collect your urine for the following 6 hours. Genova Diagnostics (Intestinal Permeability Assessment) includes the drink mix, whereas Doctor's Data (Intestinal Permeability) does not, which requires you to obtain the drink mix from your physician by prescription.

- **SIBO Breath Test (also known as Bacterial Overgrowth of the Small Intestine Breath Test)** – This test measures the amount of hydrogen and methane gases coming into the breath from the small intestine. It requires from 6 to 8 breath samples taken over a period of 2 to 3 hours after drinking a lactulose or glucose solution. Most providers prefer lactulose solution as it will not be absorbed at all and can check for SIBO throughout the entire small intestine. Glucose will absorb in and around the first 3 feet of the small intestine. Therefore, this test will only show results for this first section of the small intestine. Genova Diagnostics (Small Intestinal Bacterial Overgrowth) uses and provides the lactulose solution.

- **AIRE 2 Device for SIBO** – A new portable breath analyzing device is on the market for measuring hydrogen and methane molecules in your breath. It is offered by a company called FoodMarble and is called AIRE 2. The "2" is an updated version that includes the methane measurement and not just hydrogen. It communicates with an app that gives you real-time results. AIRE 2 can be found at https://foodmarble.com and is available directly for $179.00. Should you care to purchase this device, use code BWFM21 for a 15% discount graciously offered by FoodMarble specifically for my readers. This device can be used ongoing to help track your results. The AIRE 2 device can be especially helpful in determining how the intestine is reacting to certain foods, and I feel, will greatly allow practitioners to better diagnose and help treat patients suffering from SIBO.

- **Know Your Numbers** – Cholesterol, Blood Pressure, Blood Sugar- These three markers are critical numbers to know concerning metabolic health. They are also relatively easy to monitor yourself. Generally speaking, getting a check on your cholesterol numbers involves a visit to a lab for a blood draw. However, you can order cholesterol and more in-depth lipid blood tests yourself without visiting a physician through https://questdirect.questdiagnostics.com or https://www.walkinlab.com.

I would suggest purchasing a reliable home blood pressure monitor so that you can check your blood pressure periodically. Blood pressure is considered normal at 120/80 mm Hg or lower.

You can also purchase a glucose monitoring device for home use and check your fasting glucose level occasionally. Fasting glucose levels should optimally be under 90 mg/dl.

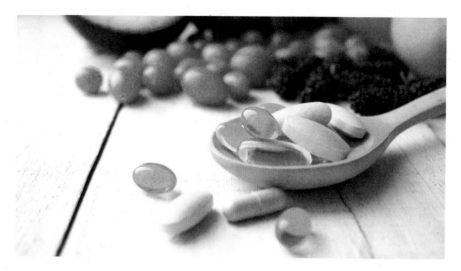

SUPPLEMENTS

The below list of supplements offers suggestions only and does not represent a formal treatment protocol. This list may not be fully inclusive for your situation. Please follow your practitioner's or doctor's suggestions, and be sure to check with your healthcare provider before starting any supplement plan.

HOPE Formula – High Fiber, Omega Oils, Probiotics, Enzymes - The HOPE Formula is a daily regimen that supports and optimizes your digestive health. Following the HOPE Formula will help you balance your gut bacteria, attain regular, satisfying bowel elimination, reduce digestive complaints, and help you digest your food more thoroughly, thereby absorbing the vital nutrients your body needs.

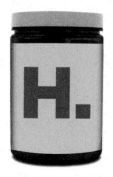

H = HIGH FIBER:

There are two types of fiber – soluble and insoluble -, and all plant-based foods contain both in varying ratios. However, you can find fiber supplements geared towards one or the other. Soluble fiber is like the soft yellow side of a scrubber sponge, soaking up unwanted toxins and excess cholesterol as it travels through the intestinal tract. Soluble fiber is also the fiber that feeds the good bacteria in your gut and is sometimes called a prebiotic. Insoluble fiber is like the green scrubber side of the sponge, helping to sweep the colon free of debris and providing bulk to the stool. Soluble fiber dissolves in water, whereas insoluble does not and travels through the intestine in much the same form as consumed.

Fiber is a critical element of good gut health, but the average American eats only between 10 to 15 grams of fiber per day, less than half of the recommended 20 to 35 grams. The best food sources of fiber are fruits, vegetables, nuts, and seeds. I strongly recommend you get a large portion of your fiber from non-starchy vegetables and low-sugar fruits. However, it can be difficult to consume 35 grams of fiber from your diet alone. A quality fiber supplement is an easy way to help you reach that daily goal.

For general health, you can look for a fiber supplement that contains both soluble and insoluble fibers from ingredients such as flax, chia, hemp, oat, or pea and offers from 6 to 13 grams of fiber per serving. Start adding fiber slowly to your diet, building to the full serving.

A supplement with more soluble fiber is suggested for diarrhea as it helps absorb the excess liquid and slows things down in the digestive tract.

A supplement geared more towards insoluble fiber content is suggested for constipation as it attracts water into your stool and ads bulk to help increase motility or movement.

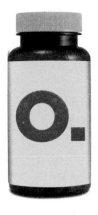

O = OMEGA-3 OILS:

According to a 2009 Harvard School of Public Health report, the 8th leading cause of death was low dietary Omega-3 intake. These vital fats are missing in many Americans' diets and drastically affect their health. Omega-3 oils are among the most well-studied nutrients and have been shown to be beneficial for cardiovascular, brain, joint, and digestive health. They play a crucial part in modulating the inflammatory response and in healing a leaky gut. The three main types of Omega-3 oils are ALA (alpha-linolenic acid), EPA (eicosapentaenoic acid), and DHA (docosahexaenoic acid).

Good food sources of Omega-3 oils are fish like salmon, sardines, mackerel, and anchovies, as well as walnuts, flaxseed, flaxseed oil, and avocados. Like with fiber, it is hard to get enough Omega-3s through your diet alone, so supplementation can be beneficial.

Look for an Omega-3 supplement that offers at least 1,000 mg of Omega-3 content per softgel. Make sure it is 1,000mg of the Omega content and not just 1,000 mg of fish oil. For optimal benefit, take 2-3 daily with food.

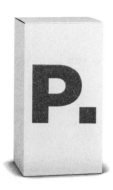

P = PROBIOTICS:

You have learned a lot about probiotics throughout this book. Hopefully, you now realize the tremendous benefit of having adequate potency and appropriate diversity of bacteria in your gut. Some probiotics can be obtained through the diet in plain yogurt, kefir, and other fermented foods but will not offer the potency or diversity your body needs.

As with fiber and omega oils, a quality probiotic supplement will give you the best opportunity to help reestablish gut health.

Look for a high potency AND high strain diversity probiotic that contains:

- At least 60 billion probiotic cultures per capsule – this is the potency
- At least 60 unique probiotic strains per capsule – this is the strain diversity
- And be sure it has both Lactobacillus and Bifidobacterium strains of bacteria!
- Prebiotics to supply food for the probiotics

Also, be sure the supplement uses some form of delayed-release technology so that the probiotic delivers the beneficial bacteria into the intestinal system and not into the stomach, where stomach acid can destroy them. With delayed-release capsules, you can take the probiotic any time of day, with or without food. Also, make sure the potency is guaranteed to end of expiration and not only at the time of manufacture.

NOTE

If you suspect SIBO or you have an increase of symptoms such as gas, bloating, and abdominal pain when initiating a probiotic supplement - Stop. Do not include probiotics in this situation until you have eradicated the overgrowth of bacteria by following a SIBO protocol. Add probiotics back slowly and monitor symptoms.

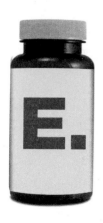

E = DIGESTIVE ENZYME:

Digestive enzymes can be beneficial for breaking down food in your stomach and small intestine. Many people find enzymes helpful for symptoms such as gas, bloating, indigestion, and heartburn.

Look for an enzyme formula that contains higher levels of at least the three essential enzymes outlined below. Take the enzymes just before eating any regular meal or with foods you know may cause you gas and bloating.

- At least 100,000 units of Protease to help break down proteins

- At least 25,000 units of Amylase to help breakdown carbohydrates
- At least 5,000 units of Lipase to help breakdown fats

In addition to the three essential enzymes, several others can be of great help at mealtime:

- **Alpha Galactosidase** – helps digest beans and legumes
- **Lactase** – helps digest lactose from dairy (make sure your enzyme has lactase if you are lactose intolerant)
- **Cellulase** – helps digest the cellulose of plant cell walls (vegetables and fruits)
- **DDP-IV** – helps digest gluten – make sure it has this if you know you are gluten intolerant (this does not include being celiac, in that case, you must avoid gluten in the diet)
- **Betaine HCl** – helps increase stomach acidity for proper digestion of protein foods
- **Pepsin** – enzyme found in combination with HCl for proper protein digestion

NOTE If you are especially sensitive to lactose or gluten, you can find those specific enzymes by themselves in a more potent dosage.

INTESTINAL SUPPORT PRODUCT

L-GLUTAMINE:

Glutamine is the most abundant amino acid in the body. It has a role in maintaining muscle integrity and performs a critical role in supporting the integrity of the intestinal lining. It is a key ingredient used by the intestinal cells, helping them to reproduce correctly. Glutamine helps regulate the strong tight junctions within the gut lining so that increased permeability is less likely (leaky gut). It is also involved in suppressing the pro-inflammatory pathway within the intestinal system. Unfortunately, glutamine stores in the body become depleted during stress, trauma, inflammatory bowel diseases, and muscle wasting diseases.

Taking a glutamine supplement during times of stress, digestive concerns, and other health issues can prove beneficial. Look for a powder supplement that offers 6,000 mg of L-glutamine per scoop.

Additional ingredients that can complement the intestinal benefit of glutamine and may be found in a supplement intended for gut health include:

- **N-Acetyl-glucosamine** – an ingredient used to produce the protective mucus which lines the intestinal tract.
- **Aloe Vera Extract** - helps coat, protect, and soothe the intestine, similar to how it soothes a sunburn on the outer skin.

- **DGL** – Deglycyrrhizinated Licorice is a licorice extract that has removed the component that can raise blood pressure. DGL stimulates the healing of damaged mucus membranes, including the stomach and intestine.

- **Ginger Root** – helps relieve indigestion and stomach upset.

- **Marshmallow Root** – helps to soothe irritation and inflammation in the intestinal tract.

NATURAL LAXATIVE FORMULA:
Although the point is to get to the root cause of occasional constipation, it can be helpful and offer more immediate relief to take a natural laxative formula. Look for one that contains ingredients such as:

- **Magnesium Hydroxide** – categorized as an osmotic laxative, it draws water into the bowel to soften stool and stimulate intestinal motility producing bowel elimination.

- **Cape Aloe Leaf** - a species of aloe from the South Africa Cape region containing natural laxative compounds.

- **Rhubarb Root** – also contains natural laxative properties and helps tone the bowel.

- **Slippery Elm** – the inner bark of the Slippery Elm tree forms a mucilage substance that can help soothe irritation and assist in bowel elimination.

- **Marshmallow Root** – also very soothing to the intestinal system and can help with stool passage through the bowel.

- **Triphala** – an Ayurvedic herbal remedy consisting of the fruits of three individual plants: Emblica officinalis, also known as Amla or Indian gooseberry, Terminalia bellirica, and Terminalia chebula. Triphala is high in antioxidants and has many health benefits in the body. It is most noted for its use in digestive issues and constipation.

SACCHAROMYCES BOULARDII – S. boulardii is a yeast organism first discovered in 1923 by French scientist Henri Boulard. It functions as a beneficial organism within the human microbiome and has been shown to offer protection against pathogenic microbes such as Clostridium difficile and the parasite Blastocystis hominis. It has also been clinically effective against antibiotic-associated diarrhea (AAD). Practitioners often recommend S. boulardii in combination with high diversity, high potency probiotics for digestive issues such as SIBO/SIFO, C. difficile, and parasitic infections.

SIBO/SIFO CLEANSE/DETOX – while trying to eradicate SIBO/SIFO, it is beneficial to take a product designed to help your body do just that. This type of product should combine several ingredients that demonstrate antibacterial properties. Keep in mind this will not further disrupt your intestinal environment but rather help in reestablishing balance. Look for a product that includes:

- **Oregano Oil** – contains a compound called carvacrol that has been shown helpful in eradicating misplaced bacteria in the small intestine.

- **Thyme Oil** – has been shown to have antifungal, antibacterial, and anti-inflammatory properties.
- **Clove Leaf Oil** – has been reported to inhibit the growth of mold, yeasts, and bacteria biofilm as well as enhance the production of our protective intestinal mucus.
- **Black Cumin Seed Oil** – has many incredible health benefits, including strong antifungal properties.
- **Cinnamon Leaf Oil** – has been demonstrated to be an effective antibacterial agent even against antibiotic-resistant bacteria.

During this process, it is helpful to look for a product that also offers liver support with such ingredients as N-Acetyl Cysteine, L-Methionine, Milk Thistle, Quercetin, Artichoke, Dandelion, and Alpha Lipoic Acid.

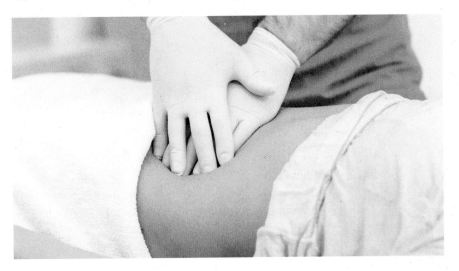

ALTERNATIVE THERAPIES

COLON HYDROTHERAPY – Colon hydrotherapy involves the process of introducing warm water under gentle pressure into the large intestine through the rectum and then relieving the pressure, stimulating a gentle release of intestinal content. The intention behind this practice is to assist the body in cleansing accumulated toxins and waste. This comfortable and hygienic process is used by many to relieve occasional constipation, give general health support, and improve overall well-being. Colon hydrotherapy can also be used to prepare for a colonoscopy procedure. Be sure you visit a colon hydrotherapist certified by the International Association of Colon Therapists (I-ACT) and is well versed in this alternative practice. You can locate someone in your area at the I-ACT website: https://www.i-act.org

Although not specific to gut health many other alternative therapies can be beneficial for stress relief and support general health and well-being. These can include massage, yoga, chiropractic care, acupuncture, meditation, tai chi, and spiritual pursuits.

REFERENCE

CHAPTER 1
A Great Extinction is Happening in YOUR GUT!

1. https://asm.org/Articles/2019/November/Disappearance-of-the-Gut Microbiota-How-We-May-Be -

2. Sonnenburg ED, Smits SA, Tikhonov M, Higginbottom SK, Wingreen NS, Sonnenburg JL. Diet-induced extinctions in the gut microbiota compound over generations. *Nature*. 2016;529(7585):212-215.

3. https://microsetta.ucsd.edu/about/american-gut-project/

4. Sonnenburg ED, Smits SA, Tikhonov M, Higginbottom SK, Wingreen NS, Sonnenburg JL. Diet-induced extinctions in the gut microbiota compound over generations. *Nature*. 2016;529(7585):212-215.

5. https://www.ted.com/talks/dan_knights_how_we_study_the_microbes living_in_your_gut/transcript?language=en

CHAPTER 2
What Causes LOMD?

1. Neu J, Rushing J. Cesarean versus vaginal delivery: long-term infant outcomes and the hygiene hypothesis. *Clin Perinatol*. 2011;38(2):321-331.

2. https://www.nichd.nih.gov/health/topics/breastfeeding/conditioninfo benefits

3. https://my.clevelandclinic.org/health/articles/15274-the-benefits-of-breastfeeding-for-baby--for-mom

4. *Front. Microbiol.*, 12 January 2016 https://doi.org/10.3389/fmicb.2015.01543

5. https://med.stanford.edu/news/all-news/2017/08/hunter-gatherers-seasonal-gut-microbe-diversity-loss.html

6. https://www.npr.org/sections/goatsandsoda/2017/08/24/545631521/is-the-secret-to-a-healthier-microbiome-hidden-in-the-hadza-diet

7. https://www.bb536.jp/english/basic/basic02.html

8. Mitsuoka T. Intestinal flora and human health. *Asia Pac J Clin Nutr*. 1996 Mar;5(1):2-9.

9. https://www.millionmarker.com/human-exposome

10. https://pubmed.ncbi.nlm.nih.gov/2044337/

11. https://www.ncbi.nlm.nih.gov/pmc/articles/PMC6829383/

12. https://www.medicalnewstoday.com/articles/320264#Differences-between-lean,-obese-subjects

13. *Hindawi Oxidative Medicine and Cellular Longevity* Volume 2017, Article ID 3831972, 8 pages http://dx.doi.org/10.1155/2017/3831972

14. https://www.medicalnewstoday.com/articles/how-gut-microbes-contribute-to-good-sleep

15. https://www.ncbi.nlm.nih.gov/pmc/articles/PMC3047904/

16. https://www.ncbi.nlm.nih.gov/pmc/articles/PMC7332307/

CHAPTER 3
Diversity and the Microbiome

https://www.ted.com/speakers/rob_knight

CHAPTER 4
CAN WE TALK?
Quorum Sensing and the Gut

1. Bonnie Bassler's TED talk - https://www.ted.com/talks/bonnie_bassler_how_bacteria_talk?language=en

2. Definition of quorum - https://languages.oup.com/google-dictionary-en/

3. Miller MB, Bassler BL. Quorum sensing in bacteria. *Annu Rev Microbiol.* 2001;55:165-99.

4. Definition of quorum sensing - https://pubmed.ncbi.nlm.nih.gov/11544353/#:~:text=Quorum%20sensing%20is%20the%20regulation,a%20function%20of%20cell%20density.

5. Wu L, Luo Y. Bacterial Quorum-Sensing Systems and Their Role in Intestinal Bacteria-Host Crosstalk. *Front Microbiol.* 2021 Jan 28;12:611413.

6. Biofilm Chandki R, Banthia P, Banthia R. Biofilms: A microbial home. *J Indian Soc Periodontol.* 2011;15(2):111-114. doi:10.4103/0972-124X.84377

CHAPTER 5
First Signs of LOMD

1. Gas - Steven R. Peikin, MD, *Gastrointestinal Health*, Quill, 1999, p. 89.

2. Diarrhea
Li Y, Xia S, Jiang X, Feng C, Gong S, Ma J, Fang Z, Yin J, Yin Y. Gut Microbiota and Diarrhea: An Updated Review. *Front Cell Infect Microbiol.* 2021 Apr 15;11:625210.

3. Constipation
Zhao and Yu *SpringerPlus* (2016)5:1130 DOI 10.1186/s40064-016-2821-1 "Intestinal microbiota and chronic constipation."

4. Archaea
   Gaci N, Borrel G, Tottey W, O'Toole PW, Brugère JF. Archaea and the human gut: new beginning of an old story. *World J Gastroenterol.* 2014;20(43):16062-16078.

CHAPTER 6
IBS - COULD IT BE MORE?
SIBO/SIFO/GERD

1. SIBO - *Miller LS, Vegesna AK, Sampath AM, Prabhu S, Kotapati SK, Makipour K. Ileocecal valve dysfunction in small intestinal bacterial overgrowth: a pilot study. *World J Gastroenterol.* 2012;18(46):6801-6808.

CHAPTER 7
LOMD - Long-term Consequences
of Inflammation

1. Cani PD, Bibiloni R, Knauf C, Waget A, Neyrinck AM, Delzenne NM, Burcelin R. Changes in gut microbiota control metabolic endotoxemia-induced inflammation in high-fat diet-induced obesity and diabetes in mice. *Diabetes.* 2008 Jun;57(6):1470-81.

2. https://www.tfah.org/report-details/state-of-obesity-2020/ - adults

3. https://www.beckershospitalreview.com/public-health/childhood-obesity-rates-hit-all-time-high-survey-finds.html

4. Ley RE, Bäckhed F, Turnbaugh P, Lozupone CA, Knight RD, Gordon JI. Obesity alters gut microbial ecology. *Proc Natl Acad Sci U S A.* 2005 Aug 2;102(31):11070-5.

5. Ley RE, Turnbaugh PJ, Klein S, Gordon JI. Microbial ecology: human gut microbes associated with obesity. *Nature.* 2006 Dec 21;444(7122):1022-3.

6. Turnbaugh PJ, Hamady M, Yatsunenko T, Cantarel BL, Duncan A, Ley RE, Sogin ML, Jones WJ, Roe BA, Affourtit JP, Egholm M, Henrissat B, Heath AC, Knight R, Gordon JI. A core gut microbiome in obese and lean twins. *Nature.* 2009 Jan 22;457(7228):480-4.

7. Turnbaugh PJ, Ley RE, Mahowald MA, Magrini V, Mardis ER, Gordon JI. An obesity-associated gut microbiome with increased capacity for energy harvest. *Nature.* 2006 Dec 21;444(7122):1027-31.

8. Bäckhed F, Ding H, Wang T, Hooper LV, Koh GY, Nagy A, Semenkovich CF, Gordon JI. The gut microbiota as an environmental factor that regulates fat storage. *Proc Natl Acad Sci U S A.* 2004 Nov 2;101(44):15718-23.

9. Kalliomäki M, Collado MC, Salminen S, Isolauri E. Early differences in fecal microbiota composition in children may predict overweight. *Am J Clin Nutr*. 2008 Mar;87(3):534-8.

10. Musso G, Gambino R, Cassader M. Obesity, diabetes, and gut microbiota: the hygiene hypothesis expanded? *Diabetes Care*. 2010 Oct;33(10):2277-84.

11. Collado MC, Isolauri E, Laitinen K, Salminen S. Distinct composition of gut microbiota during pregnancy in overweight and normal-weight women. *Am J Clin Nutr*. 2008 Oct;88(4):894-9.

12. Kershaw EE, Flier JS. Adipose tissue as an endocrine organ. *J Clin Endocrinol Metab*. 2004 Jun;89(6):2548-56.

13. Curtiss LK. Reversing atherosclerosis? *N Engl J Med*. 2009 Mar 12;360(11):1144-6.

14. Krack A, Sharma R, Figulla HR, Anker SD. The importance of the gastrointestinal system in the pathogenesis of heart failure. *Eur Heart J*. 2005 Nov;26(22):2368-74.

15. Grundy SM. Inflammation, hypertension, and the metabolic syndrome. *JAMA*. 2003 Dec 10;290(22):3000-2.

CHAPTER 8
Simple Solutions

References are inserted as resources within the chapter.